Understanding Clinical Papers Second Edition

David Bowers
School of Medicine, University of Leeds, UK

Allan House
School of Medicine, University of Leeds, UK

David Owens
School of Medicine, University of Leeds, UK

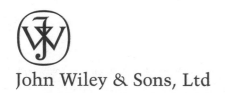

John Wiley & Sons, Ltd

Copyright © 2006   John Wiley & Sons Ltd, The Atrium, Southern Gate, Chichester,
West Sussex PO19 8SQ, England

Telephone   (+44) 1243 779777

Email (for orders and customer service enquiries): cs-books@wiley.co.uk
Visit our Home Page on www.wileyeurope.com or www.wiley.com

Other Wiley Editorial Offices

John Wiley & Sons Inc., 111 River Street, Hoboken, NJ 07030, USA

Jossey-Bass, 989 Market Street, San Francisco, CA 94103-1741, USA

Wiley-VCH Verlag GmbH, Boschstr. 12, D-69469 Weinheim, Germany

John Wiley & Sons Australia Ltd, 42 McDougall Street, Milton, Queensland 4064, Australia

John Wiley & Sons (Asia) Pte Ltd, 2 Clementi Loop #02-01, Jin Xing Distripark, Singapore 129809

John Wiley & Sons Canada Ltd, 22 Worcester Road, Etobicoke, Ontario, Canada M9W 1L1

Wiley also publishes its books in a variety of electronic formats. Some content that appears in print may not be available in
electronic books.

Library to Congress Cataloging-in-Publication Data

Bowers, David, 1938 - Understanding clinical papers / David Bowers, Allan House, David Owens. – 2nd ed.
   p. ; cm.
Includes bibliographical references and index.
ISBN 0-470-86809-0 (hardback : alk. paper) – ISBN 0-470-09130-4 (pbk. : alk. paper)
   1. Medical literature.   2. Medical writing.   3. Journalism, Medical.
      [DNLM: 1. Journalism, Medical. 2.   Reading. 3.   Writing. WZ 345 B786u 2006]
I. House, Allan. II. Owens, David, Dr. III. Title.
R118.6.B69 2006
808′.06661–dc22   2005035001

British Library Cataloguing in Publication Data

A catalogue record for this book is available from the British Library

ISBN -13 978-0-470-09130-2
ISBN-10 0-470-09130-4

Typeset in 10/12pt Times Roman by Thomson Press (India) Limited, New Delhi, India
Printed and bound in Great Britain by Antony Rowe, Ltd, Chippenham, Wiltshire
This book is printed on acid-free paper responsibly manufactured from sustainable forestry in which at least two trees are planted
for each one used for paper production.

Contents

Preface to the First Edition

Buy this book if you are a healthcare professional and you want some guidance in understanding the clinical research literature. It is designed to help you with reading research papers, by explaining their structure and the vocabulary they use. These essential first steps will make interpretation of clinical research that much easier for you. For example, the book will help with questions like:

- 'Who were the authors, what is their standing, and can they be trusted?'
- 'What question or questions did they want to answer, and what was the clinical importance of doing so?'
- 'Who were the subjects in the study, how were they chosen, and were the methods used the most suitable?'
- 'How were the data collected? Was this the best approach?'
- 'What methods did the authors use to analyse the data, and were the methods employed appropriate?'
- 'What did they find? Were their conclusions consistent with their results?'
- 'Were there any shortcomings in the study? Do the authors acknowledge them?'
- 'What are the clinical implications of their results?'
- 'Does it all make sense?'

This book is *not* an introduction to medical statistics, study design, epidemiology, systematic reviews, evidence-based medicine, or critical appraisal, although we inevitably touch on all of these things (and more). Even so, if you are not already well versed in some of these fields, you should know a lot more by the time you get to the end.

We have concentrated on improving our readers' understanding of *quantitative* research papers; and while qualitative papers contain several important elements which we have not been able to cover here, there are many other areas, particularly at the beginning and end of papers, which readers of qualitative papers will find relevant to their needs.

Primarily, this book should be of interest to the following individuals:

- Clinicians currently practising. This includes GPs, doctors in hospitals, in the community and in public health, nurses, midwives, health visitors, health educators and promoters, physiotherapists, dietitians, chiropodists, speech therapists, radiographers, pharmacists, and other clinically-related specialists.
- Clinicians of all types engaged in research activities: as part of their training; as a condition of their clinical duties; for postgraduate studies and courses; or for professional qualifications.
- Those involved with the education and training of health professionals in colleges of health, in universities, and in inhouse training and research departments.
- College, undergraduate, and postgraduate students in all medical and clinical disciplines which involve any element of research methods, medical statistics, epidemiology, critical appraisal, clinical effectiveness, evidence-based medicine, and the like.

In addition, this book should appeal to individuals who, although not themselves clinicians, nonetheless find themselves in a clinical setting and need some understanding of what the published clinical research in their area means:

- Clinical auditors and quality sensors.
- Clinical managers.
- Service managers, administrators and planners.
- Those working in health authorities and in local government social and health departments.
- Purchasers of health provision.
- People not actually employed in a clinical arena but who nonetheless have a professional or personal interest in the medical literature – for example, members of self-help and support groups; medical journalists; research-fund providers; the educated, interested, lay public.

We have structured the contents of the book into a series of chapters or units whose sequence mirrors that of papers in most of the better-quality journals. Thus we start with the preliminaries (title, authors, institution, journal type and status, and so on) and end with the epilogue (discussion, conclusions and clinical implications). Throughout the book we have used a wide variety of extracts from recently published papers to illuminate our textual comments. In these we have focussed largely, but not solely, one example of *good* practice in the hope that this will provide readers with some 'how it should be done' benchmarks. Any errors remain, of course, our own.

David Bowers, Allan House, David Owens
Leeds, 2001

Preface to the Second Edition

We received a great many favourable comments from those who used the first edition of this book–for which, many thanks. Why, then, a second edition? The reason is the usual one in these circumstances – we think we can make the book even better. When we set out to write the first edition, we had a good idea of what we wanted to include, but inevitably there was some jostling for the available space. In the end, some things that we might have included had to be left on the cutting room floor. With this second edition we have now been able to include most of that excluded material. We have also taken the opportunity to respond to some helpful suggestions from readers. In addition to these changes, we have now added a considerable amount of completely new material.

Thus, this second edition includes a new chapter on measurement scales, and new or significantly expanded sections on the following: ethical considerations; abstracts; consent to randomization into trials; pragmatic and explanatory trials; intention-to-treat analysis; elements of probability; data transformation; non-parametric tests; systematic review; among others.

Moreover, there is a lot of new material in the chapters on regression – including more on variable selection and model building, and on Cox regression. A good deal of the material in the middle chapters of the book has been re-arranged and improved to make for a better and more lucid flow (the treatment of dummy variables has been brought forward a chapter, for example).

We have all taken the opportunity to update many of the extracts from clinical papers which we use to illustrate the various ideas and procedures we describe, and also to revise much of the text in the book to improve clarity and understanding. We remain more than willing to receive any constructive comments and suggestions from readers. Otherwise we are confident that this is now an even better book than the original.

SOME NOTES ON STATISTICAL SOFTWARE

There are several statistical packages, of varying levels of sophistication and complexity, which can be used to analyse clinical data. Among the most widely used are the following:

> CIA (Confidence Interval Analysis)
> EPI-Info
> Minitab
> SPSS (the Statistics Package for the Social Sciences)
> STATA
> S-PLUS

In our opinion, Minitab is the simplest and friendliest statistics package for the general user. SPSS is not quite as easy to use but handles cross-tabulation of two variables rather better and has a wider range of the more sophisticated types of analyses. The choice of types of analysis and their outputs are perhaps easier to understand in Minitab than in SPSS. Each application has, of course, its limitations. To the best of our knowledge, Minitab does not do the McNemar test, nor does it have a clinically-based survival analysis program, nor does it allow for a direct calculation of Spearman's correlation coefficient (the data need first to be ranked). On the other hand, SPSS does not allow a chi-squared test to be done directly on a contingency table in the columns of the data sheet, nor does it Provide confidence intervals for the difference between two proportions, or with the Mann-Whitney or Wilcoxon tests, all of which Minitab does. But as we have said, SPSS has a wider range of applications.

CIA, as its name implies only does confidence interval calculations (but in this respect is very useful). EPI-Info is a combination database and epidemiological tool, which originates from the Center for Disease Control (CDC) in the USA. It has the advantage of being free (it can be downloaded from the Internet along with a user's manual).

Most professional clinical statisticians will probably use either STATA or S-PLUS; both more powerful and versatile than either Minitab or SPSS (but rather less easy to use).

We would not recommend Excel as a statistics program since it is fundamentally a spreadsheet tool and thus has an extremely limited range of statistical functions – and in any case, these are not set out in a way that is well suited to clinical research.

WRITING PAPERS FOR CLINICAL JOURNALS

Those of you who envisage writing up your research and submitting paper to a clinical journal may find the following web site addresses (URLs) useful. They contain detailed advice and instructions to authors on what is required prior to submission: for example, how to contact the journal, what should be in the paper (order and content of sections), information on the required style, editorial policies and guidelines, and so on.

The first URL directs you to a set of instructions to authors for each of over 3500 health and life-sciences journals, worldwide. The second and third URLs relate specifically to the *British Medical Journal*, but contain a huge amount of detailed and splendidly informative material related to the preparation and submission of clinical papers, and collectively provide a set of desirable standards to which anyone who is contemplating the submission of such a paper to the BMJ or any other journal should aspire:

http://mulford.mco.edu/instr
http://bmj.bmjournals.com/advice
http://bmj.bmjjournals.com/advice/article_submission.shtml

David Bowers, Allan House, David Owens,
School of Medicine, University of Leeds, Autumn, 2005

Acknowledgements

The authors and publisher wish to thank the copyright holders of the material quoted in the figures of this publication for giving their permission to reproduce the items listed below from those works, full details of which may be found in the references:

Am J Epidemiology, de Boer et al. (1998), Figure 23.1 p. 160, Haelterman *et al.* (1997), Figure 24.3 p. 171, Jernström and Olssan (1997), Figure 22.5 p. 156, McKeown-Eyssen *et al.* (2000), Figure15.6 p. 102, Olson *et al.* (1997), Figure 22.4 p. 156, reproduced by permission of Oxford University Press.

Arch Intern Med, Groenewoud *et al.* (2000), Figure 30.1 p. 218, Lien & Chan (1985), Figure 11.7 p. 72, reproduced by permission of the American Medical Association.

Arch Pediatr Adol Med, Brent *et al.* (1995), Figure 6.1 p. 35, reproduced by permission of the American Medical Association.

BMJ, Appleby *et al.* (1997), Figure 7.1 p. 46 and Figure 8.2 p. 51, Basso *et al.* (1997), Figure 17.3 p. 110, Beral *et al.* (1999), Figure 28.3 p. 204, Bhagwanjee *et al.* (1997), Figure 2.5 p. 12 and Figure 2.6 p.13, Blatchford *et al.* (1997), Figure 28.2 p. 203, Brandon *et al.* (1984), Figure 13.3 p. 84, Bruzzi *et al.* (1997), Figure 18.1 p. 114, Coste *et al.* (1994), Figure 12.4 p. 80, Cousens *et al.* (1997), Figure 7.3 p. 48, Dupuy *et al.* (1999), Figure 28.4 p. 205, Egger & Davey Smith (1998), Figure 26.3 p. 187, English *et al.* (1997), Figure 19.2 p. 124, Fahey *et al.* (1998), Figure 26.6 p. 191, Gaist *et al.* (2000), Figure 30.3 p. 220, Graham *et al.* (2000), Figure 2.2 p. 9, Grant *et al.* (2000), Figure 28.5 p. 206 and Figure 28.6 p. 207, Griffin (1998), Figure 26.5 p. 190, Grun *et al.* (1997), Figure 19.5 p. 128 and Figure 20.1 p. 131, He *et al.* (1994), Figure 23.2 p. 161, Judge & Benzeval (1993), Figure 20.2 p. 132, Kremer *et al.* (2000), Figure 28.7 p. 208, Kroman *et al.* (2002), Figure 29.7 p. 215, Levene (1992), Figure 4.4 p. 23, Little *et al.* (1997), Figure 21.2 p. 141, Macarthur *et al.* (1995), Figure 5.4 p. 32, Moore *et al.* (1998), Figure 26.4 p. 189, Murray *et al.* (1997), Figure 19.4 p. 126, Naumberg *et al.* (2000), Figure 13.4 p. 85, Oliver *et al.* (1997), Figure 14.2 p. 80, Pinnock *et al.* (2003), Figure 6.6 p. 41, Piscane *et al.* (1996), Figure 18.2 p. 115, Platt *et al.* (1997), Figure 8.1 p. 50, Poulter *et al.* (1999), Figure 2.3 p. 10, Premawardhena *et al.* (1999), Figure 6.2 p. 37 and Figure 6.4 p. 39, Reidy *et al.* (1998), Figure 28.1 p. 202, Salmon *et al.* (1998), Figure 5.2 p. 29, Singer & Freedman (1992), Figure 4.3 p. 22, Smith *et al.* (1995), Figure 11.5 p. 70, Tang *et al.* (1998). Figure 26.1 p. 184, Wald *et al.* (1997), Figure 17.4 p. 111, reproduced by permission of BMJ Publishing Group.

Br J General Practice, Little (1998), Figure 22.3 p. 154, Rodgers & Miller (1997), Figure 11.6 p. 71, reproduced with permission of the Royal College of General Practitioners.

Br J Psychiatry, Cooper *et al.* (1987), Figure 4.6 p. 25, Evans *et al.* (1999), Figure 3.3 p. 17, Figure 8.3 p. 52 and Figure 30.2 p. 219, Hawton *et al.* (1997), Figure 16.1 p. 108, reproduced by permission of the Royal College of Psychiatrists.

Brain, Tebartz van Elst *et al.* (2000), Figure 3.2 p. 16, reproduced by permission of Oxford University Press.

Clinical Chemistry, Van Steirteghem *et al.* (1982), Figure 14.1 p. 88, Reproduced by permission of AACC.

Cochrane Database of Systematic Reviews, Gibbs *et al.* (2005), fig 26.2, p.185, reproduced by permission of the Cochrane Library.

Geriatric Nursing, Culbertson *et al.* (2004), Figure 4.5 p. 24, Ellenbecker *et al.* (2004) Figure 4.7 p. 26, reproduced by permission of Elsevier Science.

International Journal of Epidemiology, Grandjean *et al.* (2000), Figure 24.2 p. 168, reproduced by permission of Oxford University Press.

J Advanced Nursing, Hagen *et al.* (2003), Figure 15.4 p.100, Figure 15.5 p. 101, and Figure 15.8 p.104, Hundley *et al.* (2000), Figure 10.3 p. 60, Kong (2005), Figure 2.1 p. 8, Lin *et al.* (2005), Figure 21.5 p. 144 and Figure 25.2 p. 179, Miles *et al.* (2002), Figure 15.1 p. 94 and Figure 15.7 p.103, reproduced by permission of Blackwell Science.

J Am Med Assoc, Topol *et al.* (1997), Figure 11.3 p. 67 and Figure 21.3 p. 142, reproduced by permission of the American Medical Association.

J Clinical Nursing, Ho & Lopez (2003), Figure 15.3 p. 96, Farnell *et al.* (2005), Figure 23.3, p.163, reproduced by permission of Blackwell Science.

J Epidemiol Commun Health, Lindelow *et al.* (1997), Figure 14.3 p. 91, Peabody & Gertler (1997), Figure 11.4 p. 69, reproduced by permission.

J Neurol Psychiatry, Carson *et al.* (2000), Figure 7.2 p. 47, reproduced by permission.

Lancet, Adams *et al.* (1999), Figure 29.9 p. 216, Adish *et al.* (1999), Figure 9.2 p. 55, Chosidow *et al.* (1994), Figure 11.2 p. 67, Cooper *et al.* (1999), Figure 6.5 p. 40, Criqui & Ringel (1994), Figure 5.1 p. 28, Dunne *et al.* (1999), Figure 27.3 p. 196, Emerson *et al.* (1999), Figure 29.3 p. 212, Feeney *et al.* (1997), Figure 5.3 p. 31, Goldhaber *et al.* (1999), Figure 29.8 p. 216, Hancox *et al.* (2003), Figure 24.5 p. 175, Kwakkel *et al.* (1999), Figure 29.1 p. 210, Lacy *et al.* (2002), Figure 21.6 p. 145 and Figure 27.4 p.198, Ledergerber *et al.* (1999), Figure 29.6 p. 214, Mansi *et al.* (1999), Figure 27.2 p. 195, Marshall *et al.* (1995), Figure 13.1 p. 81 and Figure 13.2 p. 82, MERIT-HF Study Group (1999), Figure 29.2 p. 211, Möttönen *et al.* (1999), Figure 29.5 p. 213, Nikolajsen *et al.* (1998), Figure 12.2 p. 78 and Figure 19.3 p. 125, Singh & Crockard (1999), Figure 29.4 p. 212, Søyseth *et al.* (1995), Figure 12.3 p. 79 and Figure 21.4 p. 143, Taylor *et al.* (1999), Figure 18.3 p. 118, Thompson *et al.* (2000), Figure 2.4 p. 11 and Figure 3.1 p. 15, Turnbull *et al.* (1996), Figure 21.7 p. 147, Unwin *et al.* (1999), Figure 10.2 p. 59, all copyright The Lancet Ltd, reproduced by permission of Elsevier Science.

Nature Medicine, Long *et al.* (2000), Figure 1.1 p. 3 and Figure 1.3 p. 6, reproduced by permission.

Neurology, Rogers *et al.* (1998), Figure 9.1 p. 54 and Figure 13.5 p. 86, copyright 1998, reproduced by permission of Lippincott, Williams & Wilkins (a Wolters Kluwer Company).

New Engl J Medicine, Michelson *et al.* (1996), Figure 19.1 p. 123 and Figure 21.1 p. 194, Pollack *et al.* (2002), Figure 27.1 p. 194. Copyright Massachusetts Medical Society. All rights reserved. Reproduced by permission.

Pediatrics, Nead *et al.* (2004), Figure 25.3 p. 180, Phipatanakul *et al.* (2004), Figure 25.1 p. 178, reproduced by permission of the American Association of Pediatricians.

Quality in Health Care, Hearn & Higinson (1999), Figure 15.2 p. 95, McKee & Hunter (1995), Figure 22.2 p. 153, reproduced by permission.

Stroke, Henderson *et al.* (2000), Figure 1.2 p. 4, reproduced by permission.

Venereology, Ho Han *et al.* (1999), Figure 10.1 p. 57, reproduced by permission.

I

Setting the Scene:
Who Did What, and Why

1

Some Preliminaries

Before you start reading a paper, you could usefully ask one or two questions which help set the work in context. Here they are:

WHO WROTE THE PAPER?

Often, one person writes an article such as a review or an editorial. This is less common for papers describing the results of a research study. Because most research is a joint enterprise, papers describing research studies are usually published under the names of a number of people – the research team. From the list of authors, you can tell:

- *the range of expertise of the research team.* Professional backgrounds of the authors (and sometimes their level of seniority) are often included, with the address of each.
- *the research centre or centres involved in the study.* This is useful when you've been reading for a while and you know whose work to look out for – for whatever reason!
- *the principal researcher.* He or she is often named first, or sometimes identifiable as the only author whose full address and contact details are listed (called the corresponding author).

Figure 1.1 shows a typical example of a research project which required a collaborative effort.

Gender differences in HIV-1 diversity at time of infection

E. Michelle Long, Harold L. Martin, Jr, Joan K. Kriess,
Stephanie M. J. Rainwater, Ludo Lavreys, Denis J. Jackson, Joel Rakwar,
Kishorchandra Mandaliya & Julie Overbaugh

Division of Human Biology, Fred Hutchinson Cancer Research Center, Seattle, Washington, USA
Molecular and Cellular Biology program, Departments of Microbiology,
Medicine and Epidemiology, University of Washington, Seattle, Washington, USA
Department of Medical Microbiology, University of Nairobi, Nairobi, Kenya.
Correspondence should be addressed to J.O.: email: joverbau@fhcrc.org

This project involved workers from several disciplines . . .

. . . the corresponding author is listed last rather than, as is often the case, first . . .

. . . the work came from research centres in two countries.

FIGURE 1.1   Authors and research centres listed at the head of a research article

---

Understanding Clinical Papers Second Edition   David Bowers, Allan House, David Owens
© 2006 John Wiley & Sons, Ltd

The list of authors may be quite long. The more people involved with a study, the less likely it is that one of them has a pre-eminent position, so there may be no principal author. The authors may simply be listed in alphabetical order.

When a large study involving many sites is published, it may be that the work is written up by a small team, on behalf of the larger group. You may then find that there are no named authors, or only one or two, and the rest of the team is listed elsewhere – as in Figure 1.2. This type of multiple authorship is unavoidable if everybody is to get credit for participating in large studies.

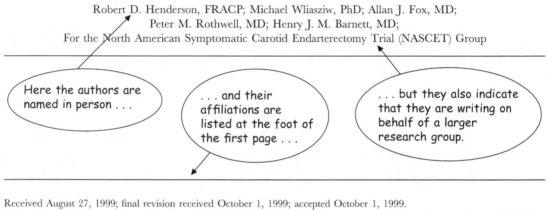

Angiographically Defined Collateral Circulation and Risk of Stroke in Patients with Severe Carotid Artery Stenosis

Robert D. Henderson, FRACP; Michael Wliasziw, PhD; Allan J. Fox, MD;
Peter M. Rothwell, MD; Henry J. M. Barnett, MD;
For the North American Symptomatic Carotid Endarterectomy Trial (NASCET) Group

Received August 27, 1999; final revision received October 1, 1999; accepted October 1, 1999.
From the John P. Robarts Research Institute (R.D.H., M.E., H.J.M.B.) and Departments of Epidemiology and Biostatistics (M.E.), Clinical Neurological Sciences (M.E., A.J.F., H.J.M.B.), and Diagnostic Radiology (A.J.F.), University of Western Ontario, London, Ontario, Canada; and Department of Clinical Neurology, Radcliffe Infirmary, Oxford, UK (P.M.R.).
Correspondence to H.J.M. Barnett MD, John P. Robarts Research Institute, 100 Perth Dr, PO Box 5015, London, Ontario N6A5K8, Canada, E-mail barnett@rri.on.ca

FIGURE 1.2   Authorship on behalf of a large research group

An undesirable form of multiple authorship arises if members of an academic department attach their names to a paper when they had nothing to do with the study. This is sometimes called 'gift authorship', although it isn't always given very freely. To try to stop this practice, many journals now expect each author to explain exactly what part he or she has played in the study. For this, and other useful information, you should turn to the *acknowledgements* at the end of the paper.

IN WHAT SORT OF JOURNAL DOES THE PAPER APPEAR?

Not all journals are the same. Some are mainly aimed at members of a particular professional group, and therefore include political news, commentaries, and personal opinions. Others publish only research articles which have not appeared elsewhere, while some aim to mix these functions.

In some journals, the letters pages are designed to allow readers to express their opinions about articles which have appeared in previous issues. In others, the letters pages contain only descriptions of original studies.

What appears in a journal is decided by the editor, nearly always with the help and advice of an editorial committee. The best journals also seek opinions from external referees who comment on papers sent to them, and advise on suitability for publication. Because these referees are usually experts in the same field as the authors of the paper, this process is called 'peer reviewing'. It isn't always easy to tell whether papers for a journal are peer-reviewed, which is unfortunate because the peer-reviewing process is the best means of establishing the quality of a journal's contents. You shouldn't trust the results of any data-containing study if it appears in a journal which does *not* use the peer-reviewing system.

Some journals produce *supplements*, which are published in addition to the usual regular issues of the main journal. They may be whole issues given over to a single theme, or to describing presentations from a conference or symposium. Often they are produced (unlike the main journals) with the help of sponsorship from pharmaceutical companies. Papers in these supplements may not have been reviewed by the same process as papers in main journals, and for that reason they tend not to be of as high quality.

One way to judge the quality of a journal is to check its *impact factor* – a measure of the frequency with which papers in the journal are quoted by other researchers.[*] The impact factor is only a rough guide because high quality journals that cover very specialized topics will inevitably have lower ratings than journals with a wider readership.

WHO (AND WHAT) IS ACKNOWLEDGED?

It is tempting to treat the acknowledgements at the end of a paper as being a bit like the credits after a film – only of interest to insiders. But they contain interesting information. For example, who's credited with work, but doesn't feature as an author? This is often the fate of medical statisticians and others who offer specialist skills for the completion of one task in the study. If the study required special expertise – such as advanced statistics, economic analysis, supervision of therapists – then the necessary 'expert' should be a member of the research team and acknowledged. If not, then either the expert wasn't a member of the team, or somebody isn't getting credit where it's due. To ensure that co-authorship is earned, and to guard against research fraud, the acknowledgements in many journals now also contain a statement from each author about his or her individual contribution.

The acknowledgements section from the first paper we looked at showed what additional help the research team received (see Figure 1.3). It also contains an indication of the *source of funding* that supported the research. This is of interest because external funding *may* bring with it extra safeguards as to the rigour with which work was conducted. On the other hand, it may lead to a *conflict of interest* – for example, if a pharmaceutical or other commercial company has funded research into one of its own products.

Declaring a conflict of interest is *not* the same as admitting to a guilty secret. Its aim is to ensure that readers, when they are making their judgements about the study, are informed that there may be non-scientific influences on the conduct or interpretation of a study.

_____

[*]You can check the impact factor of a journal at a number of websites including (for example) the ISI Journal Citation Reports. These are available through many Health Science libraries and web sites.

Gender differences in HIV-1 diversity at time of infection

E. Michelle Long, Harold L. Martin, Jr, Joan K. Kriess,
Stephanie M. J. Rainwater, Ludo Lavreys, Denis J. Jackson, Joel Rakwar,
Kishorchandra Mandaliya & Julie Overbaugh

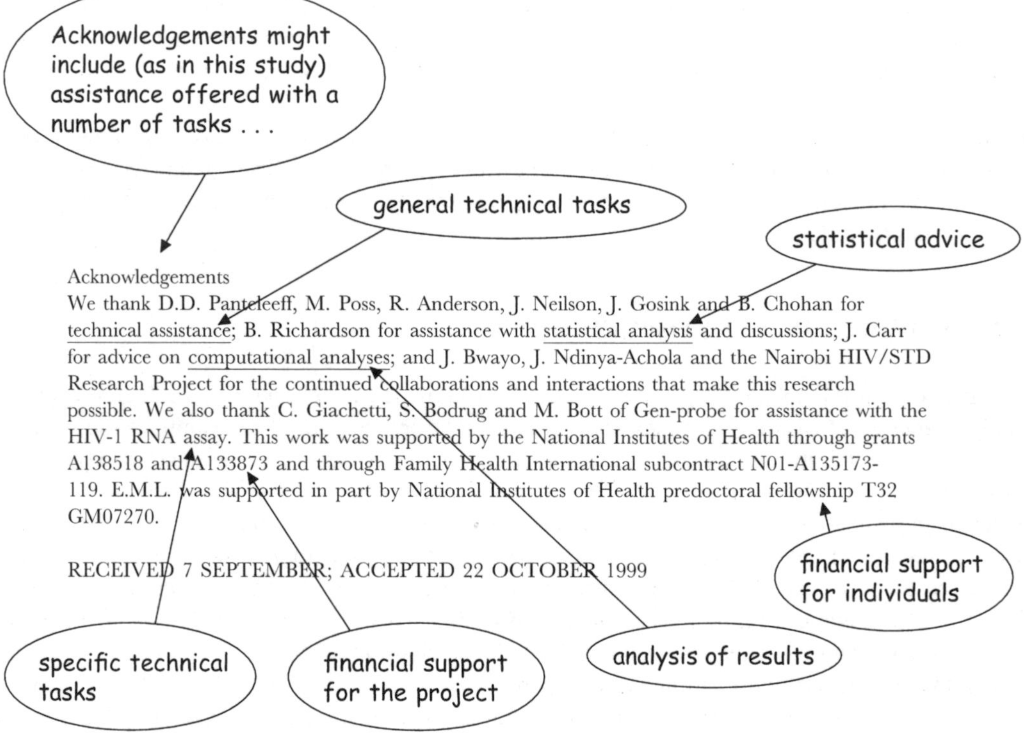

FIGURE 1.3   Acknowledgement of statistical, financial and other support at the end of a paper

2

The Abstract and Introduction

If the title of an article doesn't give you a clear enough idea of what it's about, then most papers reporting primary research data start with an abstract – a brief summary of the whole paper that appears immediately below the title.

THE ABSTRACT

The purpose of this brief summary is to help the reader decide if they want to go on to read the paper in detail, by outlining the content of the research and its main findings. A good abstract should help the reader decide – if this study has been well conducted, then is it one about which I would be interested enough to read further?

Some journals require authors to provide structured abstracts – using headings equivalent to those that appear in the main text. A typical example is shown in Figure 2.1. Other abstracts are unstructured and simply give a brief narrative account of the accompanying paper. The decision about which style of abstract to use is determined not by the author but by the journal.

THE INTRODUCTION

After the abstract comes an introductory section. Its aim is to provide some background information that makes it clear why the study described in the paper has been undertaken. The general topic area of the paper may be very familiar, but even so (perhaps especially so) the authors will probably give some summary of its importance, possibly along the lines of:

- Is it clinically important? Is it about a symptom that affects quality of life, or causes major treatment difficulties?
- Is there a public health importance? Is it about an illness that represents a big burden for the community – in terms of chronic handicap, or costs to health or social services?
- Is the interest theoretical? Will further study help us to understand the causes of a condition, or its consequences?

Figure 2.2 shows the introduction to a study which examined the effect of two ways of presenting information to women who were making decisions about antenatal testing.

These questions will normally be discussed by *reference to existing evidence*. The Introduction to a paper is not the place to look for a comprehensive literature review, and introductory sections in most papers are brief, but there are one or two pointers to help you decide if the evidence is being presented in a fair and unbiased way:

- Is there reference to a systematic review (see Chapter 26)? Or if not, to a search strategy which the authors used to identify relevant evidence? For an example, see Figure 2.3.

Understanding Clinical Papers Second Edition   David Bowers, Allan House, David Owens
© 2006 John Wiley & Sons, Ltd

Day treatment programme for patients with eating disorders: randomized controlled trial

Seongsook Kong

Aim This paper reports a randomized controlled trial to compare the effects of day treatment programmes for patients with eating disorders with those of traditional outpatient treatment.

Background Eating disorders are common, especially in adolescents, and their worldwide prevalence is increasing. Treatment interventions for patients with eating disorders have traditionally been offered on an outpatient or inpatient basis, but the recent introduction of day hospital programmes offers the possibility of greater cost-effectiveness and relapse-prevention for this population.

Methods Volunteers from an outpatient clinic for eating disorders were randomly assigned either to a treatment group ($n = 21$), participating in a modified day treatment programme based on the Toronto Day Hospital Program, or to a control group ($n=22$) receiving a traditional outpatient programme of interpersonal psychotherapy, cognitive behaviour therapy and pharmacotherapy. Data were collected from January to December 2002 using the Eating Disorder Examination, Eating Disorder Inventory-2, Beck Depression Inventory, and Rosenberg Self-Esteem Scale.

Results Participants in the day treatment programme showed significantly greater improvements on most psychological symptoms of the Eating Disorder Inventory-2, frequency of binging and purging, body mass index, depression and self-esteem scores than the control group. They also showed significant improvement in perfectionism, but the group difference was not significant.

Conclusion Nurses in day treatment programmes can play various and important roles establishing a therapeutic alliance between patient and carer in the initial period of treatment. In addition, the cognitive and behavioural work that is vital to a patient's recovery, that is, dealing with food issues, weight issues and self-esteem, is most effectively provided by a nurse therapist who maintains an empathic involvement with the patient.

Keywords Day treatment, depression, eating disorders, nursing, outcome, self-esteem

A structured abstract uses headings also found in a full paper.

Some abstracts give actual results, others summarize the main findings.

FIGURE 2.1 An example of a structured abstract – this one from a trial of two treatment programmes for patients with eating disorders

- Is the evidence mainly from the authors' own group, or do the authors quote a range of evidence, even if it is not in support of their own views?
- Many clinical studies are carried out because the evidence is ambiguous or contradictory. Is there a dilemma which is posed by the evidence, and is it clearly spelled out in the Introduction?

Randomised controlled trial comparing effectiveness of touch screen with leaflet for providing women with information on prenatal tests

Wendy Graham, Pat Smith, A Kamal, A Fitzmaurice, N Smith, N Hamilton

Introduction

Informed choice has been an important component of health care in the United Kingdom for almost a decade. One area in which this principle has long been applied is prenatal testing. Specific initiatives have been launched to promote women's awareness of best evidence on the effectiveness of specific tests and active participation in decisions about their care. The number of conditions for which screening is offered continues to grow rapidly, and women consequently face increasingly complex decisions. Studies have illuminated many dimensions to this complexity, including the professional and organisational barriers to informed choice, the huge variations in the scope and accuracy of information given, and the problem of receiving unsolicited and unanticipated information from screening. What is also clear is that informed choice depends on an effective partnership between the user, the provider and the communication medium.

Throughout the NHS, efforts are being made to evaluate traditional methods of conveying information, such as leaflets, and to develop and assess new approaches. This paper reports the results of a recent trial to evaluate a touch screen information system for providing information on prenatal tests to women.

> The authors start by emphasizing the difficulty for women in exercising informed choice in a complex area.

> They go on to indicate the role of communication in making that choice easier . . .

> . . . and they point to the increased interest in evaluating new ways of helping people make choices.

FIGURE 2.2   Explaining the background to a research study

Generally speaking, the justification for a new study is that the existing evidence is unsatisfactory, and a typical Introduction summarizes why, as in Figure 2.4. The commonest justifications for new research are that:

- Different studies have come to different conclusions about the topic, and it isn't possible to come to an answer without new work.
- The evidence cannot be applied in the setting being considered by the authors. For example, good evidence may cease to be of value simply because it is old – trials showing the benefit of treatment may no longer be useful if a disorder changes so that its sensitivity to treatment changes. Similarly, evidence from one part of the world cannot always be applied freely elsewhere.
- The evidence may be incomplete. For example, we may know that rates of smoking are increasing among young women but we don't know why.
- The evidence may be of poor quality, so that no conclusion can be drawn from it (Figure 2.4).

Association between birth weight and adult blood pressure in twins: historical cohort study

N R Poulter, C L Chang, A J MacGregor, H Snieder, T D Spector

Introduction

A meta-analysis of 34 studies has shown a significant inverse relation between birth weight and subsequent levels of blood pressure. Compared with higher birthweight babies, low birthweight babies have been shown to have higher levels of blood pressure as children, adolescents, and adults, the association being more pronounced with age. It is hypothesised that some adverse aspect or aspects of intrauterine life, such as nutritional deficiencies at critical periods of fetal growth, programme the fetus to have higher levels of blood pressure after birth. The mechanisms invoked to produce this programming effect include the impact of impaired fetal growth on blood vessel growth or compliance or the number of nephrons.

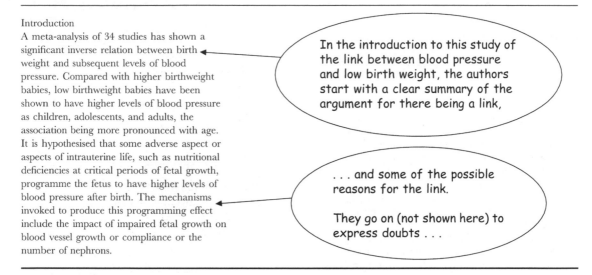

In the introduction to this study of the link between blood pressure and low birth weight, the authors start with a clear summary of the argument for there being a link,

. . . and some of the possible reasons for the link.

They go on (not shown here) to express doubts . . .

FIGURE 2.3 Meta-analytic review quoted in a paper's introduction

If these elements of the introduction are well presented, then it should be clear what the paper is about, and why the authors have chosen to conduct the work that they have. Armed with this background briefing, you can now move on to check the *specific objectives* of the authors' work.

ETHICAL CONSIDERATIONS

Nearly all studies in healthcare that involve contact with people will require ethical approval. What that means is that the researchers will have had to submit their proposals to a panel of experts, such as a local research ethics committee, who decide whether the project is ethical or not. For example, the risks of any research should be outweighed by its benefits, and participants should have been given the opportunity to participate or not as they wished, without their decision influencing their medical care.

Most authors will indicate that their study has been approved by the appropriate body governing research ethics – usually either in the methods section or the acknowledgements. Increasingly, authors will mention any particular ethical dilemmas raised by their research either in the introduction or the discussion of their paper. Where there are particular questions raised by a study, the authors may expand upon them – including, for example, details of the information given to participants and the way in which consent was obtained.

Certain types of research cause particular ethical concerns. For example, young children, or those with cognitive impairment or learning disability, or patients who are unconscious, cannot give consent to participate in research that nonetheless asks extremely important questions about clinical care. In these situations, researchers may undertake research with ethical approval, provided certain criteria are met (see Figure 2.5 and the commentary in Figure 2.6).

Effects of a clinical-practice guideline and practice-based education on detection and outcome of depression in primary care: Hampshire Depression Project randomised controlled trial

C Thompson, A L Kinmonth, L Stevens, R C Peveler, A Stevens, K J Ostler, R M Pickering, N G Baker, A Henson, J Preece, D Cooper, M J Campbell

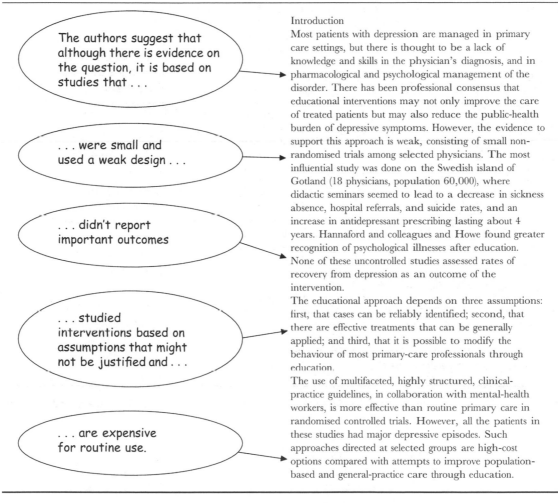

The authors suggest that although there is evidence on the question, it is based on studies that . . .

. . . were small and used a weak design . . .

. . . didn't report important outcomes

. . . studied interventions based on assumptions that might not be justified and . . .

. . . are expensive for routine use.

Introduction

Most patients with depression are managed in primary care settings, but there is thought to be a lack of knowledge and skills in the physician's diagnosis, and in pharmacological and psychological management of the disorder. There has been professional consensus that educational interventions may not only improve the care of treated patients but may also reduce the public-health burden of depressive symptoms. However, the evidence to support this approach is weak, consisting of small non-randomised trials among selected physicians. The most influential study was done on the Swedish island of Gotland (18 physicians, population 60,000), where didactic seminars seemed to lead to a decrease in sickness absence, hospital referrals, and suicide rates, and an increase in antidepressant prescribing lasting about 4 years. Hannaford and colleagues and Howe found greater recognition of psychological illnesses after education. None of these uncontrolled studies assessed rates of recovery from depression as an outcome of the intervention.

The educational approach depends on three assumptions: first, that cases can be reliably identified; second, that there are effective treatments that can be generally applied; and third, that it is possible to modify the behaviour of most primary-care professionals through education.

The use of multifaceted, highly structured, clinical-practice guidelines, in collaboration with mental-health workers, is more effective than routine primary care in randomised controlled trials. However, all the patients in these studies had major depressive episodes. Such approaches directed at selected groups are high-cost options compared with attempts to improve population-based and general-practice care through education.

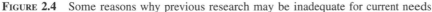

FIGURE 2.4   Some reasons why previous research may be inadequate for current needs

Does HIV status influence the outcome of patients admitted to a surgical intensive care Unit? A prospective double blind study

Satish Bhagwanjee, David JJ Muckart, Prakash M Jeena, Prushini Moodley

Introduction

Limited resources and the high cost of intensive care have compelled clinicians to rationalise the allocation of resources. For example, in our unit it is policy not to admit patients with incurable malignant disease, and end-stage liver disease, and patients with multiple organ failure who are deemed non-salvageable. The lack of objective data made it unclear whether patients with HIV infection should be treated similarly. To allow rationalisation of the admissions policy with respect to these patients we conducted a prospective study to determine the prevalence of HIV infection among patients admitted to the unit and assess the impact of HIV status (HIV positive, HIV negative, AIDS) on outcome. The study embraced a major ethical dilemma. On the one hand, the clinician has an obligation of non-maleficence – that is, patients must not be harmed by the actions of the doctor. On the other hand, the doctor has an obligation to society to ensure that available resources are appropriated fairly, based on objective evidence. Though the basic ethical tenets of patient autonomy, justice, beneficence, and non-maleficence are useful, they are only the starting points for ethical decision making.

Subjects and methods The study was conducted in the 16 bed surgical intensive care unit at King Edward VIII Hospital, a large teaching hospital in Durban. All patients admitted to the unit over six months (September 1993 to February 1994) were included. There were no exclusions. Informed consent was not sought. The study protocol was approved by the ethics committee of the University of Natal.

This research studied a topic identified by the authors as being of great ethical importance ...

... implicitly, the ethical importance of the work was taken to justify the inclusion of non-consenting (unconscious) patients.

FIGURE 2.5   Discussion of ethical considerations from a study into the outcomes of surgical patients and their HIV status

Commentary: Why we did not seek informed consent before testing patients for HIV

Satish Bhagwanjee, David JJ Muckart, Prakash M Jeena, Prushini Moodley

Commentary We agree completely with the Nuremberg code and the Helsinki declaration that informed consent is an essential prerequisite for medical research. However, we believe that there may be extraordinary circumstances when this right may be waived. We identify four crucial requirements that must be fulfilled before research without informed consent may be permitted.

Requirements that must be satisfied before research without consent

1. It is impossible to obtain informed consent. Eighty-five per cent of admissions to our unit are emergency cases. These patients cannot give informed consent because they are critically ill. A second option is to obtain consent from a relative. In our study this would have resulted in two possible scenarios.

The journal's editors thought the ethical challenge so great that they invited a more extensive discussion to accompany the paper.

FIGURE 2.6   Commentary on the paper from which Figure 2.5 is taken

3

The Objectives

Following the Introduction, you should look for a clear statement of the *objectives* of the current work. This statement can come in two forms: the aims of the study and the hypotheses to be tested.

- *Aims* are general statements about purpose. For example, the authors might wish to examine the attitudes of hospital nurses to colleagues with mental health problems.
- *Hypotheses* are specific questions, suggested by previous research or theory. For example, does taking the oral contraceptive pill increase the risk of stroke among women of childbearing age?

HYPOTHESES

Often, studies will ask more than one question, in which case they will have several hypotheses. In these circumstances, you should look for a *main hypothesis* (see Figures 3.1 and 3.2), and the other questions will form *subsidiary or secondary hypotheses*.

There are important reasons why a study should have only one main question:

- If a study tests many hypotheses, then just by chance it is likely to produce positive results for some of them. (See Chapter 21 on hypothesis testing and the possibility of false positive results from *multiple testing*.)

Effects of a clinical-practice guideline and practice-based education on detection and outcome of depression in primary care: Hampshire Depression Project randomised controlled trial

C Thompson, A L Kinmonth, L Stevens, R C Peveler, A Stevens, K J Ostler, R M Pickering, N G Baker, A Henson, J Preece, D Cooper, M J Campbell

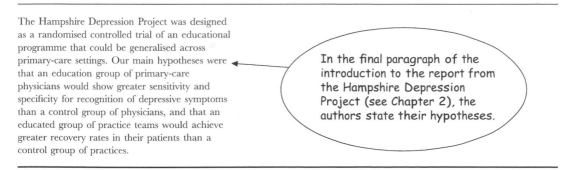

The Hampshire Depression Project was designed as a randomised controlled trial of an educational programme that could be generalised across primary-care settings. Our main hypotheses were that an education group of primary-care physicians would show greater sensitivity and specificity for recognition of depressive symptoms than a control group of physicians, and that an educated group of practice teams would achieve greater recovery rates in their patients than a control group of practices.

In the final paragraph of the introduction to the report from the Hampshire Depression Project (see Chapter 2), the authors state their hypotheses.

FIGURE 3.1   Statement of a study's main hypothesis

Understanding Clinical Papers Second Edition   David Bowers, Allan House, David Owens
© 2006 John Wiley & Sons, Ltd

Affective aggression in patients with temporal lobe epilepsy: A quantitative MRI study of the amygdala

L. Tebartz van Elst, F.G. Woermann, L. Lemieux, P.J. Thompson and M.R. Trimble

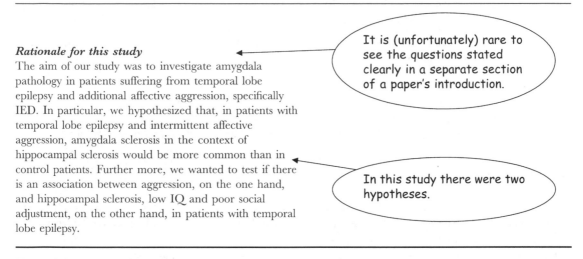

Rationale for this study

The aim of our study was to investigate amygdala pathology in patients suffering from temporal lobe epilepsy and additional affective aggression, specifically IED. In particular, we hypothesized that, in patients with temporal lobe epilepsy and intermittent affective aggression, amygdala sclerosis in the context of hippocampal sclerosis would be more common than in control patients. Further more, we wanted to test if there is an association between aggression, on the one hand, and hippocampal sclerosis, low IQ and poor social adjustment, on the other hand, in patients with temporal lobe epilepsy.

It is (unfortunately) rare to see the questions stated clearly in a separate section of a paper's introduction.

In this study there were two hypotheses.

FIGURE 3.2   A study with two hypotheses

- We can trust a negative result only if we know that a study was large enough, otherwise, there is a possibility of false negative results. Many researchers therefore make an *estimate of sample size* to help them decide how big to make their study so that they can avoid this sort of error (see Chapter 8). To do that calculation they need to know what the *main outcome* of interest is, and the main outcome will be chosen to test the main hypothesis.

There used to be a conventional way of stating a study's hypothesis, which involved the use of a *null hypothesis*, and the description of a study set up to *disprove or refute an hypothesis*. Although this approach is still sometimes taught, you will almost never come across examples in papers. The null hypothesis was a way of stating a question in the form 'situation A is no different from situation B'. It arose because certain statistical tests operate by testing whether an assumption of similarity is likely to be true.

The need to refute rather than prove an hypothesis is similarly based on a technical point – about the nature of scientific evidence. In fact, nearly everybody now states their hypotheses in a straightforward way. The English doesn't have to be difficult to follow for the science to be right!

Not all questions are framed as hypotheses. For example, in a study examining the rate of antibiotic resistance among postoperative wound infections the authors might have no definite rate in mind.

HYPOTHESIS GENERATION

Not all studies are designed to test hypotheses – some are designed to generate new ideas and questions for future research. This is especially true of qualitative research.

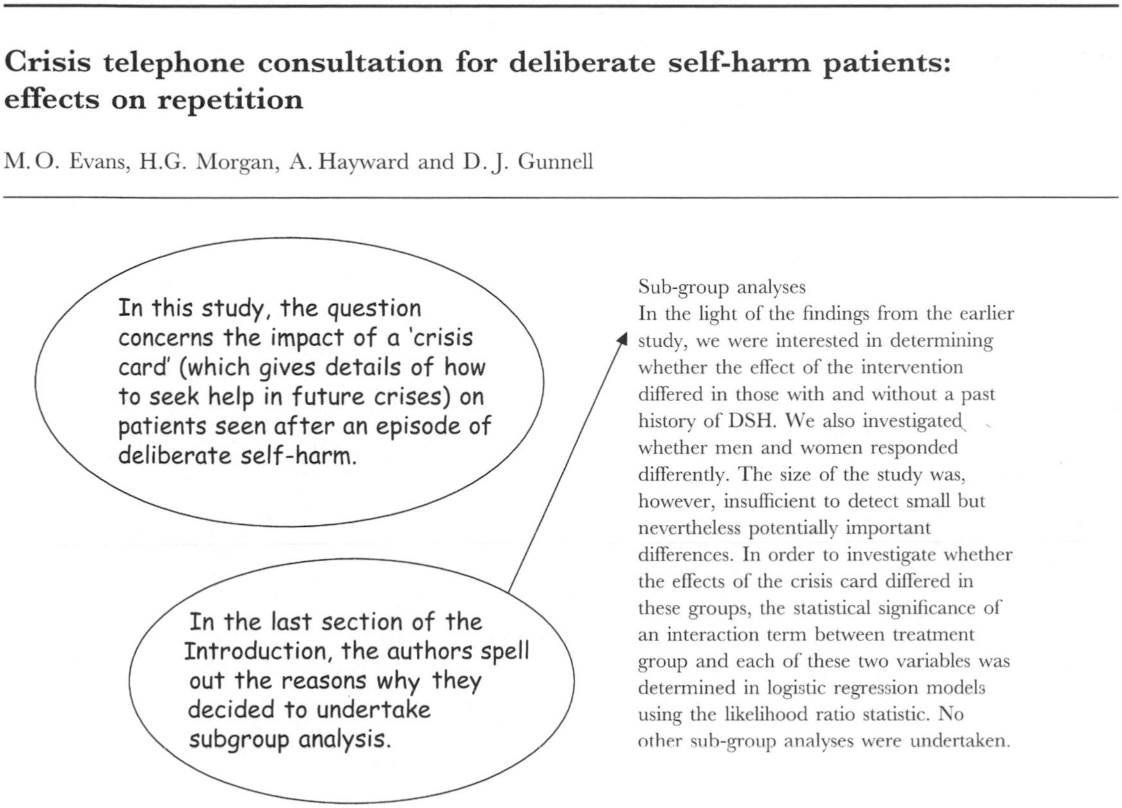

Crisis telephone consultation for deliberate self-harm patients: effects on repetition

M. O. Evans, H.G. Morgan, A. Hayward and D. J. Gunnell

In this study, the question concerns the impact of a 'crisis card' (which gives details of how to seek help in future crises) on patients seen after an episode of deliberate self-harm.

In the last section of the Introduction, the authors spell out the reasons why they decided to undertake subgroup analysis.

Sub-group analyses
In the light of the findings from the earlier study, we were interested in determining whether the effect of the intervention differed in those with and without a past history of DSH. We also investigated whether men and women responded differently. The size of the study was, however, insufficient to detect small but nevertheless potentially important differences. In order to investigate whether the effects of the crisis card differed in these groups, the statistical significance of an interaction term between treatment group and each of these two variables was determined in logistic regression models using the likelihood ratio statistic. No other sub-group analyses were undertaken.

FIGURE 3.3 Subgroup analysis used to explore possible associations which were not sought as part of the study's original hypotheses

Sometimes hypotheses are generated by subgroup analysis and *post hoc* examinations of the data produced by quantitative research (see Figure 3.3). Hypothesis generation of this sort should be regarded as unreliable but interesting. Be careful to look out for this, because some authors present these as established results rather than ideas for future work.

If you cannot find a mention of the study's objectives expressed as aims or hypotheses, you may yet be able to find them expressed in less clear-cut ways. Examples include 'exploring associations' or (worse) 'examining issues'. You will need to be particularly careful about studies with such vague objectives: because they are not asking a specific question it is not easy to tell whether the results are meaningful or whether they could have been produced by chance – especially as a result of multiple testing.

II

Design Matters:
What Type of Study are you Reading About?

4

Descriptive Studies

As you read a research paper, the next important question to ask is: What sort of study did the authors undertake? Broadly speaking, quantitative research may be either *observational* or *experimental*. In the first, the researcher actively observes patients by doing things like asking questions and taking samples; the researcher does not experiment with the patient's treatment or care. In a typical experimental study, in contrast, the researcher intervenes to ensure that some or all of a group of people receive a treatment, service or experience.

It can be helpful to divide observational studies into two groups according to their complexity (Figure 4.1). *Descriptive* studies ask questions like: What are the clinical or biochemical characteristics of people who have rheumatoid arthritis? How common a condition is asthma? How disabled do people become over a decade of follow-up after a diagnosis of multiple sclerosis? Other observational studies compare groups to try to answer more complex questions: Do people who smoke get more heart disease than those who don't smoke? Are women who experienced venous thrombosis more likely to have been taking the oral contraceptive pill than women who didn't sustain a thrombosis? Studies that ask these kinds of non-experimental (observational) questions, but that involve comparisons, are often described as *analytic*.

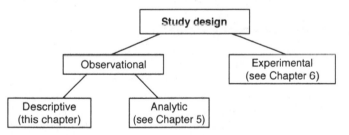

FIGURE 4.1   Types of research study design

Analytic observational studies are dealt with in Chapter 5 and experimental studies in Chapter 6. The remainder of this chapter tackles the simplest forms of observation – descriptive studies. We find it useful to subdivide descriptive studies into four types (see Figure 4.2).

CASE REPORTS

Some would say that case reports are scarcely research at all. They usually take the form of an unusual clinical case with something about the cause or the outcome of the person described that the author hopes will intrigue you. Perhaps the author's care over detail – eliciting symptoms, possible precipitants and treatments offered – takes the case report out of the ordinary clinical arena and justifies the title of research. Research journal editors vary in their views; some publish such reports and others do not.

Understanding Clinical Papers Second Edition   David Bowers, Allan House, David Owens
© 2006 John Wiley & Sons, Ltd

Types of descriptive research

Case reports

Case series

Cross-sectional studies*

Longitudinal studies

* simple cross-sectional studies determining, for example, how common (prevalent) a condition is. More complex cross-sectional studies involving comparisons are dealt with under analytic research (Chapter 5).

FIGURE 4.2   Types of descriptive research

CASE SERIES

A respectable form of research is a description of clinical findings seen in a succession of patients who seem to display a similar condition: the case series. Something unexpected has turned up – more cases than usual of a rare disorder perhaps, or an apparent excess of some clinical sign – hence the motive for writing-up the series of cases. For example, Figure 4.3 shows how clinicians used a case series to point to the dangers of playing around on bouncy castles.

Injuries sustained on "bouncy castles"

Gian Singer, Lawrence S Freedman

SIR,—We wish to report the dangers of playing on "bouncy castles." A bouncy castle is an inflatable children's playground, consisting essentially of a rubber mattress inflated with air. Three walls generally surround the castle, with the fourth side open to allow entry and exit, but some castles are open on all four sides. They are popular in fairgrounds and recreational halls. During last summer five children and one adult were treated at Northwick Park Hospital for injuries sustained while they were playing on bouncy castles. All injuries were to the arm or neck.

Three supracondylar fractures of the humerus occurred. Two of these required open reduction and internal fixation with Kirschner wires. The third was managed with a collar and cuff support. A girl aged 6 sustained a fracture of the mid-shaft of the humerus, which was managed with a hanging cast support. The neck injuries occurred in a 52 year old man and a 12 year old boy. These were both soft tissue injuries caused by flexion and were managed conservatively.

The authors noticed an unexpectedly high number of attendances at the hospital due to injuries sustained whilst playing on inflatable castles . . .

. . . and perhaps bouncy castle injuries are usually to the arm or neck, and are especially likely to be supracondylar fractures of the humerus.

FIGURE 4.3   Extract from case series of bouncy castle injuries

Sometimes the author of a case series notices some common feature that the cases share and speculates that this factor might help to explain the condition. A famous example of such studies includes the early descriptions of the birth abnormalities that became linked with the drug thalidomide.

CROSS-SECTIONAL STUDIES

Unlike the case series which usually reports an unexpected clinical encounter, the researchers of a cross-sectional study deliberately set out to assemble a group of study subjects – often patients in current or recent contact with part of the health service – and describe the presence and absence of various clinical features. For example, responding to the case series of bouncy castle injuries (Figure 4.3), another researcher extracted from a national survey of leisure accidents the clinical and circumstantial details of 105 bouncy castle injuries (see Figure 4.4) – providing us with a more representative picture.

More injuries from "bouncy castles"

S Levene

SIR,—In response to Gian Singer and Lawrence S Freedman's letter[1] I have analysed national figures for accidents involving "bouncy castles." The Department of Trade and Industry's leisure accidents surveillance system records all people injured in accidents other than home, industrial, or road traffic accidents who present to a sample of 11 hospitals throughout the United Kingdom, with 24 hour accident and emergency departments receiving at least 10 000 cases a year. One hundred and five such people were recorded, suggesting a national estimate of roughly 4000 people injured severely enough for them to present to hospital.

Thirty people were injured by falling off the castle (17 male, 13 female; five aged 0–4, 12 aged 5–9, 12 aged 10–14, and one aged 22). Parts of the body commonly injured were the foot, ankle, or toe (10 cases) and the arm, elbow, wrist, or hand (eight cases). Most injuries were minor bruising, cuts, or swelling (20 cases), but there were six fractures and three sprains or strains. Two children required admission for fractures to the arm or elbow. The locations of the bouncy castles varied: six were at fairgrounds and five at indoor sports centres.

Seventy five people were injured on the castle itself (31 male, 44 female; eight aged 0–4, 33 aged 5–9, 27 aged 10–14, and seven adults). Thirty two fell over and 14 were struck by another child, usually after the patient had fallen over. The arm, elbow, wrist, or hand (27 cases), the face and neck (nine cases), and the ankle or foot (15 cases) were commonly injured. Fifty injuries were minor, with nine fractures, 10 sprains and strains, and two dislocations. Fairgrounds (10 cases) were the most common site for the castle.

This author responded to publication of the case series by extracting (from data collected for a large leisure accident surveillance system) information about 105 cases of bouncy castle injury – presenting us with a cross-section study.

Because of their larger number and their systematic collection, these patients are likely to be more representative than the six people who happened to attend the hospital where the case series was based . . .

. . . and it is plain that the injuries are not only to the head and neck; there is, after all, no specific bouncy castle enjury.

FIGURE 4.4 Extract from cross-sectional study about bouncy castle injuries

Ear and hearing status in a multilevel retirement facility

Deborah S. Culbertson, Marcella Griggs and Suzanne Hudson

Abstract

The primary purpose of this study was to evaluate ear and hearing status in a retirement facility. Two measures of earwax occlusion, hearing impairment, hearing handicap, and cognitive function were made for 49 residents across a 1- to 4-month interval. Forty-nine percent of these residents had excessive or impacted earwax at time measurement #1 and 30.6% at time measurement #2. Because the other measures showed minimal change, time 1 and 2 measures were averaged, resulting in an incidence of 79.3% for moderate or greater hearing impairment, 39.0% for cognitive deficit, 12.5% for significant self-reported hearing handicap, and 17.2% for significant staff-reported handicap. A higher incidence of excessive and impacted earwax, moderate or greater hearing impairment, and cognitive deficit was found for residents in assisted living and nursing care than for residents in independent living. Recommendations for hearing impairment and handicap screening and effective communication strategies are offered.

> About half of the residents of the retirement complex were judged to have too much earwax when the study's participants were first examined.

FIGURE 4.5   Prevalence of a clinical feature, determined in a cross-sectional study

This new, premeditated study of 105 cases is a fairly typical cross-sectional study. It seems to show that, when the matter is examined using a suitably selected sample, there is no convincing evidence that bouncy castle injuries cause a specific fracture of the elbow region, but instead, lead to all manner of soft tissue, joint and bony injuries – anywhere on the body.

A particular type of cross-sectional, single-group study is one in which incidence or prevalence of a condition is determined. *Prevalence* studies determine how many cases of a condition or disease there are in a given population, or establish the frequency of a clinical finding in a study sample. For example, researchers might use hospital and pharmacy records to establish how many people have insulin-receiving diabetes in a defined hospital catchment area. Then again, another study might estimate the proportion of older people in residential facilities whose ears are occluded by earwax (see Figure 4.5).

Incidence studies are rather similar but refine the above kind of study in two ways: the incidence of a condition is the number of *new* cases arising in a defined population over a defined *time*. Figure 4.6 describes such a study – to determine in 12 cities across five continents the number of first contacts with psychiatric services arising from symptoms of a psychotic illness. The researchers established the two-year incidence (sometimes called *inception rate*) of schizophrenia in each of the cities. Strictly

The Incidence of Schizophrenia in Nottingham

J. E. COOPER, D. GOODHEAD, T. CRAIG, M. HARRIS, J. HOWAT and J. KORER

Attempts were made to identify, and include in a two-year follow-up study, every patient living in the catchment area of the Mapperley group of psychiatric hospitals in Nottingham (population 390 000) who made their first-ever contact with the psychiatric services for a potentially schizophrenic illness during a two-year period (1 August 1978 to 31 July 1980). Screening was based upon symptoms rather than diagnosis, covering both in-patient and out-patient services; a consensus diagnosis using ICD-9 was made by the project team. The Nottingham Psychiatric Case Register was used in a retrospective Leakage Study which added nine cases to the 99 identified by the screening procedures. Incidence rates are given for both broad and narrow concepts of schizophrenia, and for DSM-III diagnosis. The Nottingham incidence rates are similar to those reported from other UK centres, and are near the middle of the range found in the other collaborating centres in the WHO study on Determinants of Outcome of Severe Mental Disorders. At entry to the study, 27 patients were out-patients, and 11 were never admitted to hospital at any time in the two-year follow-up period. Reasons for believing that the Nottingham administrative incidence may be close to the incidence in the community are discussed.

The authors wanted to know about the frequency of developing schizophrenia and about its clinical features.

FIGURE 4.6   Extract from a cross-sectional (incidence) study about frequency of schizophrenia

speaking, it is this incorporation of time, as well as the proportion of cases, that makes incidence a rate while prevalence is merely a proportion (see Chapter 14). Figure 4.6 is an extract from only the Nottingham, UK, part of the multicentre study.

Some incidence and prevalence research data are derived from *case registers* – many of which have been set up with research and clinical service in mind and routinely records data useful for both purposes. In other cross-sectional studies the researchers undertake a survey of the study sample, where this survey has been set up – whether by interview, or by electronic or paper self-report – specifically for the research project. For example, researchers might ask nurses who visit patients in their homes to describe, by filling in a paper questionnaire, how their patients are using prescribed medicines (see Figure 4.7).

LONGITUDINAL STUDIES

When researchers study a group of subjects over time in a *longitudinal study*, there is more research work to be done than in a cross-sectional study; subjects must be followed up one or more times to determine their *prognosis* or *outcome*.

The kinds of observational studies we've seen above are among the simplest forms of clinical research. In the next chapter, more complex observational studies are described – *analytic* studies. What they have in common (and in this way they differ from the above study types) is that they generally involve *comparison* of two or more groups of people and often attempt to infer something about cause of symptoms or conditions.

Nurses' observations and experiences of problems and adverse effects of medication management in home care

Carol Hall Ellenbecker, Susan C. Frazier and Sharon Verney

Abstract

The purpose of this nonexperimental, descriptive study was to explore and describe the current state of medication management for patients receiving services from certified home health care agencies (CHHAs). Data were collected by self-report from a convenience sample of 101 home health care nurses from 12 agencies in six states. Nurses reported on a total of 1467 patients. Results of this study support the findings from previous research on medication management of older people living in the community. The majority of older home care patients were taking more than five prescription drugs. Many patients were taking medications in ways that deviated from the prescribed medication regimen. The results also suggest that patients are experiencing many adverse effects from medication errors. The reasons for these errors were reported to be a result of individual patient characteristics and, most frequently, communication problems in the system. Results of this study support recommendations for technology application, regulatory and policy changes, further research, and nursing practice.

Community-based nurses were given a paper survey asking them, among other things, about their patients' receipt and use of prescribed medication, for example, whether the patients were taking multiple drugs and whether they skipped doses or took the wrong amounts.

FIGURE 4.7   Use of a survey method in a cross-sectional study

5

Analytic Studies

Recall from the previous chapter that, compared with descriptive studies of a single group, analytic studies are more complex (and often more interesting). Analytic studies will usually involve some comparison and frequently aim to elucidate cause and effect in some way. Four kinds of observational study will be described here:

- ecological studies
- cross-sectional, two-group studies
- case–control studies
- cohort studies.

ECOLOGICAL STUDIES

A neat way of tackling questions about the cause of a disease is to sit in a library (or at a computer), locate routinely collected data, and put population data about disease frequency (such as regional deaths from heart disease) together with data about exposure to a risk (such as regional data on tobacco consumption). By so doing, you might find that regions with high lung cancer death rates were also the ones with high tobacco consumption. Suppose also that you found the opposite – that low mortality areas were associated with low tobacco consumption – then your findings would support a link between the supposed risk (smoking) and the target disorder (lung cancer).

The real study used as an example in Figure 5.1 concerns the 'French paradox': strikingly low mortality from coronary heart disease in France compared with other economically similar countries. Researchers from California looked into this observation by assembling data for 21 relatively wealthy countries. For each of these countries they compared the coronary heart disease mortality (taken from World Health Statistics Annuals) with the data for wine consumption (obtained from the Alcohol Research Foundation in Toronto). The extract here shows, with one of the study graphs, how the researchers use the data to shed more light on this intriguing issue about whether alcohol, and wine in particular, protects against heart disease.

But you may by now have spotted a flaw in this type of study: we don't know whether the individual people who died from heart disease were abstainers from wine. Put another way, it is possible for a study of this design to come up with these findings even if every person who died from heart disease was a heavy wine drinker. This flaw is sometimes called the *ecological fallacy* and is a consequence of the use of aggregated data rather than the more usual research method of collecting data for each individual study participant. The other three types of analytic study set out below are more satisfactory approaches to cause-and-effect questions because they are able to relate the supposed risk factor directly to the outcome in each study participant.

CROSS-SECTIONAL, TWO-GROUP STUDIES

Some cross-sectional studies aim to shed light on cause and effect by recording whether people with a disease were more likely than people without the same disease to have experienced exposure to a risk

Understanding Clinical Papers Second Edition   David Bowers, Allan House, David Owens
© 2006 John Wiley & Sons, Ltd

Does diet or alcohol explain the French paradox?

M H Criqui, Brenda L Ringel

Summary

The low rate of coronary heart disease (CHD) in France compared with other developed countries with comparable dietary intake has been called the French paradox. We explored this paradox by looking at alcohol, diet, and mortality data from 21 developed, relatively affluent countries in the years 1965, 1970, 1980, and 1988. We assessed wine, beer, and spirits intake separately.

France had the highest wine intake and the highest total alcohol intake, and the second lowest CHD mortality rate. In univariate analyses, ethanol in wine was slightly more inversely correlated with CHD than total wine volume. In multivariate analyses, animal fat tended to be positively correlated, and fruit consumption inversely correlated, with CHD. Beer and spirits were only weakly inversely correlated with CHD. The strongest and most consistent correlation was the inverse association of wine ethanol with CHD. However, wine ethanol was unrelated to total mortality.

We conclude that ethanol, particularly wine ethanol, is inversely related to CHD but not to longevity in populations. Although light to moderate alcohol

> At first sight it appears that high wine consumption might protect against heart disease.

> This graph uses the technique of correlation; plotting for each country its value for mortality against its value for wine consumption.

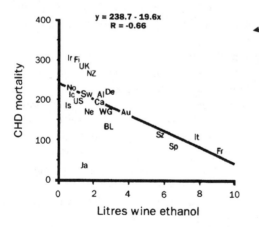

Figure 2: **Correlations of age adjusted CHD mortality rates per 100 000 with dietary items in 1988**

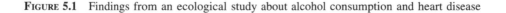

FIGURE 5.1   Findings from an ecological study about alcohol consumption and heart disease

factor. For example, for more than half a century researchers have recognized that patients with schizophrenia, when compared with the general population, are more likely to come from lower socio-economic classes. What is a lot less clear is whether lower socio-economic status is a risk factor for schizophrenia or, conversely, whether schizophrenia causes a slide down the socio-economic scale. The cross-sectional study design – in which the researcher measures in each subject a supposed risk factor at the same time as recording the presence of a condition – will nearly always have this *chicken or egg* problem (which comes first?).

In a study of bullying (Figure 5.2), the researchers persuaded 904 co-educational secondary school pupils aged 12–17 to declare whether they were bullied or not and to self-report their feelings – including a scale that measured their level of anxiety. They found that those who reported being bullied also reported more anxiety. Notice that the study design does not preclude either possibility: that bullying exacerbates anxiety or that anxious children are more likely to be targets for bullies.

It is a limitation of cross-sectional designs that the direction of any effect cannot be determined because the supposed risk factor and the outcome are identified at the same time. The next two analytic study designs tackle this issue and are able to identify the direction of any effect.

Bullying in schools: self reported anxiety, depression, and self esteem in secondary school children

G Salmon, A James, D M Smith

Variable	Being bullied or bullying	
	No	Yes
Bullied children (mean score for being bullied) $\geq$2)		
School:		
A	377	24
B	489	14
School year:		
8	224	16
9	237	8
10	194	9
11	211	5
Sex:		
Male	439	23
Female	427	15
Mean (SD) score:		
Anxiety	9.71 (6.00)	17.71 (6.75)
Esteem	29.27 (4.75)	24.97 (6.38)
Lying	2.52 (2.10)	3.37 (2.33)
Depression	5.88 (5.13)	12.92 (7.95)

Notice that bullied children have higher anxiety and depression and lower self-esteem. But is it because they are bullied, or do these characteristics lead to the bullying?

FIGURE 5.2 Extract from table of summary statistics from cross-sectional study of bullying and self-reported anxiety (values are numbers of schoolchildren unless stated otherwise)

CASE–CONTROL STUDIES

One way of avoiding the problem of cause and effect is to concentrate on a clinical scenario where the characteristic that you suspect may be a risk factor and the outcome can only have arisen in that order. Consider for a moment smoking and lung cancer: it is plain that contracting lung cancer cannot have led someone to become a long-standing heavy smoker.

Notice though that it is the pre-existence of heavy smoking that defines the difference between this example and the cross-sectional ones above. If a researcher wanted to know if high blood pressure made stroke more likely and chose to measure blood pressure in two groups of patients who were and were not victims of stroke, then any finding that hypertension was more prevalent in stroke patients might be a consequence of the stroke rather than a contributory cause. If, on the other hand, each set of patients had previously had their blood pressure recorded some years before – then the finding that stroke patients had a past excess of hypertension might very well point to high blood pressure being a risk factor for stroke.

Case–control study is the label applied to a study such as the one just mentioned, about high blood pressure and stroke. The group of people with the condition are called the *cases* and they are compared with another group who are free of the disease and are called the *controls*. The comparison to be drawn is the exposure of each of the two groups to a supposed risk factor; were the cases more often exposed to the risk than were the controls? For further discussion of cases and controls, see Chapters 9 and 10.

In the study in Figure 5.3, researchers in Dorset and York undertook a case–control study to help to settle controversy over measles vaccination in childhood and whether it predisposes to development in adulthood of inflammatory bowel disease – ulcerative colitis and Crohn's disease. They ascertained the vaccination history, from general practice records, of 140 patients with definite inflammatory bowel disease (the cases). For each of these patients they randomly selected from the same general practitioner's list two people of the same age and sex (the controls); they then ascertained the vaccination history of these control patients. They found that 79 of the 140 cases (56%) had received measles vaccine compared with 160 of the 280 controls (57%): almost exactly the same proportions. The authors conclude that their findings provide no support for the notion that measles vaccination in childhood predisposes to later development of inflammatory bowel disease.

COHORT STUDIES

Another way of identifying any relation between measles vaccine and inflammatory bowel disease would have been to compare the eventual outcome for people who were or were not vaccinated – a *cohort study*. In this hypothetical example, the subjects of the research would have been divided according to whether they were vaccinated or not. In the earlier, real, case–control study they were divided by whether they had the disease or not; the designs are quite different.

In a real example of a cohort study shown in Figure 5.4, researchers in Canada looked into whether having received epidural anaesthesia during labour is a risk factor for postpartum back pain. The subjects of study were a consecutive series of 329 women who had a child delivered at the hospital. As it happened, about half of the women had opted for epidural anaesthesia – allowing their comparison with those who had alternative forms of pain relief. A research nurse interviewed all the patients and rated on a scale their degree of self-reported pain at three follow-up points during the six weeks following delivery.

COMPARING AND CONTRASTING CASE–CONTROL AND COHORT STUDIES

Compared with cohort studies, case–control studies are cheap and cheerful. First, they can be completed without waiting for the outcome to develop. Second, there is no need for enormous numbers of study

A case-control study of measles vaccination and inflammatory bowel disease

Mark Feeney, Andrew Clegg, Paul Winwood, Jonathon Snook, for the East Dorset Gastroenterology Group

Summary

Background The cause of inflammatory bowel disease (IBD) remains to be established. Evidence has linked measles infection in early childhood with the subsequent risk of developing IBD, particularly Crohn's disease. A cohort study raised the possibility that immunisation with live attenuated measles vaccine, which induces active immunity to measles infection, might also predispose to the later development of IBD, provoking concerns about the safety of the vaccine.

Method We report a case-control study of 140 patients with IBD (including 83 with Crohn's disease) born in or after 1968, and 280 controls matched for age, sex and general practitioner (GP) area, designated to assess the influence of measles vaccination on later development of IBD. Documentary evidence of childhood vaccination history was sought from GP and community health records.

Findings Crude measles vaccination rates were 56.4% in patients with IBD and 57.1% among controls. Matched odds ratios for measles vaccination were 1.08 (95% CI 0.62–1.88) in patients with Crohn's disease, 0.84 (0.44–1.58) in patients with ulcerative colitis, and 0.97 (0.64–1.47) in all patients with IBD.

Interpretation These findings provide no support for the hypothesis that measles vaccination in childhood predisposes to the later development of either IBD overall or Crohn's disease in particular.

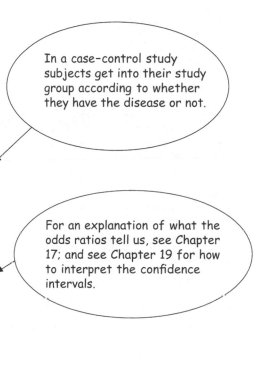

In a case-control study subjects get into their study group according to whether they have the disease or not.

For an explanation of what the odds ratios tell us, see Chapter 17; and see Chapter 19 for how to interpret the confidence intervals.

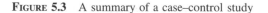

FIGURE 5.3 A summary of a case–control study

subjects who don't develop the disease. Because in a case–control study it is already clear who has the disease, only a convenient number (needed for reasonable statistical precision) of these 'controls' is needed. In a cohort study, however, there is no way of knowing who will or will not get the disease – so everyone has to be included until the study end-point reveals who has developed the condition so far. For a great many relatively uncommon outcomes the case–control study is favoured for just these reasons. Examples of case–control studies include investigating whether deep venous thrombosis is related to taking the oral contraceptive pill, and whether depressive illness is related to adverse life events and difficulties.

On the other hand, there are serious shortcomings with case–control studies. They are prone to extra biases – in particular, those concerned with recollection of past events. Suppose, for example, that a study hypothesis is that an adult condition such as motor neurone disease is predisposed to by certain kinds of childhood infections. It is likely that in an effort to understand why one has such an illness,

Epidural anaesthesia and low back pain after delivery: a prospective cohort study

Alison Macarthur, Colin Macarthur, Sally Weeks

Abstract

Objective—To determine whether epidural anaesthesia during labour and delivery is a risk factor for postpartum back pain.

Design—Prospective cohort study with follow up at one day, seven days, and six weeks after delivery.

Setting—Teaching hospital in Montreal.

Subjects—329 women who delivered a live infant(s) during the study period. Exclusion criteria were back pain before pregnancy and delivery by elective caesarean section.

Intervention—Epidural anaesthesia during labour and delivery.

Main outcome measures and results—The primary outcome variable was development of postpartum low back pain. Back pain was quantified with self reports (yes/no), a pain score (numeric rating scale), and degree of interference with daily activities. Of the 329 women, 164 received epidural anaesthesia during labour and 165 did not. The incidence of low back pain in epidural *v* non-epidural group was 53% *v* 43% on day one; 21% *v* 23% on day seven; and 14% *v* 7% at six weeks. The relative risk for low back pain (epidural *v* non-epidural) adjusted for parity, delivery, ethnicity, and weight was 1.76 (95% confidence interval 1.06 to 2.92) on day one; 1.00 (0.54 to 1.86) on day seven; and 2.22 (0.89 to 5.53) at six weeks. There were no differences between the two groups in pain scores or the frequency of interference with daily activities. Similar results were

> In a cohort study subjects get into their study group according to whether they were exposed to the supposed risk or not.

> For an explanation of what the relative risks tell us, see Chapter 17; and see Chapter 19 for how to interpret the confidence intervals.

FIGURE 5.4 Cohort analytic study examining the relation between postpartum back pain and epidural anaesthesia during labour

sufferers with motor neurone disease may recall more such illnesses than controls who have no pressure to make such an effort. It is very difficult to avoid such bias.

Second, it is usually difficult to select a wholly suitable control group for a case–control study. In a case–control study concerned with smoking and lung cancer, for example, should those without the cancer be people with other cancers, or other respiratory conditions, or other patients at the hospital without chest disorder, or general practice cases (and should they exclude those with chest problems) or members of the general public who are not drawn from healthcare contacts at all? None of these possible groups is wholly suited nor unsuited; in the end, the findings will often be hard to interpret whichever control group is selected (sometimes case–control studies use more than one control group for just such reasons).

Cohort studies avoid the worst aspects of the above two problems. First, because exposure is assessed at the start of the study, it is not subject to false remembering later. Second, assessment of exposure to risk provides sensible exposed and unexposed groups and avoids uncertainty over which comparison group to choose.

Both these two kinds of analytic observational study are greatly prone to *confounding*. This matter is discussed in Chapters 10 and 24.

6

Intervention Studies

In an American study to determine ways of improving the incidence and duration of breast-feeding (Figure 6.1), a 'lactation consultant' assisted women who were contemplating or undertaking breast-feeding. The lactation consultant saw women before and after childbirth and several times more over the

Breast-feeding in a Low-Income Population

Program to Increase Incidence and Duration

Nancy B. Brent, MD, IBCLC; Beverly Redd, IBCLC; April Dworetz, MD, MPH; Frank D'Amico, PhD; J. Joseph Greenberg, MD

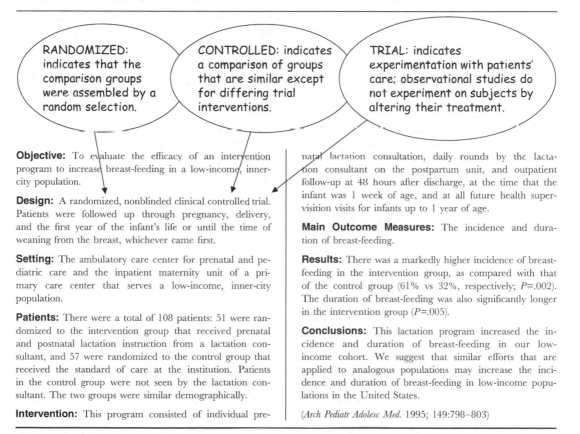

RANDOMIZED: indicates that the comparison groups were assembled by a random selection.

CONTROLLED: indicates a comparison of groups that are similar except for differing trial interventions.

TRIAL: indicates experimentation with patients' care; observational studies do not experiment on subjects by altering their treatment.

Objective: To evaluate the efficacy of an intervention program to increase breast-feeding in a low-income, inner-city population.

Design: A randomized, nonblinded clinical controlled trial. Patients were followed up through pregnancy, delivery, and the first year of the infant's life or until the time of weaning from the breast, whichever came first.

Setting: The ambulatory care center for prenatal and pediatric care and the inpatient maternity unit of a primary care center that serves a low-income, inner-city population.

Patients: There were a total of 108 patients: 51 were randomized to the intervention group that received prenatal and postnatal lactation instruction from a lactation consultant, and 57 were randomized to the control group that received the standard of care at the institution. Patients in the control group were not seen by the lactation consultant. The two groups were similar demographically.

Intervention: This program consisted of individual pre-

natal lactation consultation, daily rounds by the lactation consultant on the postpartum unit, and outpatient follow-up at 48 hours after discharge, at the time that the infant was 1 week of age, and at all future health supervision visits for infants up to 1 year of age.

Main Outcome Measures: The incidence and duration of breast-feeding.

Results: There was a markedly higher incidence of breast-feeding in the intervention group, as compared with that of the control group (61% vs 32%, respectively; *P*=.002). The duration of breast-feeding was also significantly longer in the intervention group (*P*=.005).

Conclusions: This lactation program increased the incidence and duration of breast-feeding in our low-income cohort. We suggest that similar efforts that are applied to analogous populations may increase the incidence and duration of breast-feeding in low-income populations in the United States.

(*Arch Pediatr Adolesc Med.* 1995; 149:798–803)

FIGURE 6.1 Summary of a randomized controlled trial investigating an intervention aimed at promoting and prolonging breast-feeding

next three months. In the study, about half of the 108 women who agreed to take part received the intervention; the other half did not. The mothers were randomly allocated to one or other of these groups using a procedure governed by random numbers. The outcome favoured the intervention group, both in terms of incidence and duration of breast-feeding.

TRIALS

The study depicted in Figure 6.1 has three defining features. First, it is called a *trial* because the researchers have introduced experimentation; they have arranged for some subjects but not others to receive the intervention. Second, they fix it so that their two groups of subjects will differ only according to whether or not they had the intervention. We would therefore expect, for instance, as many first-time mothers, as many affluent mothers, and as many poorly educated mothers in each of the two treatment groups. If so, none of these factors can have accounted for the difference found in outcomes; researchers often assert that these factors have been *controlled* for. But how can the groups be made similar in every way? This can happen only when allocation to one or other group is by a *randomized* procedure.

This kind of study, the *randomized controlled trial*, has become almost the only acceptable way of judging the benefit of a treatment (whether it be a drug, procedure, operation, psychological therapy or other intervention). Although it would be a lot more convenient only to investigate what happens to the treated group, the problem is that if the treated patients were to get better, it might have been for reasons unconnected with the treatment – for example, the condition might simply have resolved with time. But if, in a comparison of two similar patient groups, those who got the treatment improved more than those who didn't get it – then we have compelling evidence in favour of the treatment; improvement due to the passage of time could not explain why the treated patients had the better outcome.

In a study from Sri Lanka (extract shown in Figure 6.2), where there are many species of poisonous snakes, and venomous bites are consequently a serious health hazard, researchers used the principle of the randomized controlled trial to answer an important treatment question: Can the dangerous side-effects of life-saving anti-venom serum be counteracted?

RANDOM ALLOCATION AND ITS CONCEALMENT

Clinical trials such as the examples above often declare that treatment was allocated randomly. In recent times, though, there has been particular attention given to whether this process of randomization was scrupulously adhered to at the point of treatment allocation – by concealing the imminent allocation from the person who first administers one or other treatment.

There are several ways of determining treatment randomly. Computers can generate random numbers, or printed tables of random numbers can be referred to. Either way, the process can be carried out in advance and the results put into sealed, opaque and tamper-proof envelopes. The person who obtains the patient's consent to take part in the trial can then simply open the next envelope and proceed with the randomly allocated decision therein. Unfortunately, this admirable procedure is not beyond subversion; clinical researchers have been known to shine bright lights through envelopes to reveal the allocation, and to open several envelopes in advance of seeing potential subjects, and then allocate treatment according to their non-random judgement. A better (more tamper-proof) system is distant randomization, for example by telephone or by the internet. The researcher, after obtaining consent, calls up the randomization service, registers the index patient's entry to the study, and only then is given the answer to the random allocation.

Low dose subcutaneous adrenaline to prevent acute adverse reactions to antivenom serum in people bitten by snakes: randomised, placebo controlled trial

A P Premawardhena, C E de Silva, M M D Fonseka, S B Gunatilake, H J de Silva

Objective To assess the efficacy and safety of low dose adrenaline injected subcutaneously to prevent acute adverse reactions to polyspecific antivenom serum in patients admitted to hospital after snake bite.
Design Prospective, double blind, randomised, placebo controlled trial.
Setting District general hospital in Sri Lanka.
Subjects 105 patients with signs of envenomation after snake bite, randomised to receive either adrenaline (cases) or placebo (controls) immediately before infusion of antivenom serum.
Interventions Adrenaline 0.25 ml (1:1000).
Main outcome measures Development of acute adverse reactions to serum and side effects attributable to adrenaline.
Results 56 patients (cases) received adrenaline and 49 (controls) received placebo as pretreatment. Six (11%) adrenaline patients and 21 (43%) control patients developed acute adverse reactions to antivenom serum (P=0.0002). Significant reductions in acute adverse reactions to serum were also seen in the adrenaline patients for each category of mild, moderate, and severe reactions. There were no significant adverse effects attributable to adrenaline.
Conclusions Use of 0.25 ml of 1:1000 adrenaline given subcutaneously immediately before administration of antivenom serum to patients with envenomation after snake bite reduces the incidence of acute adverse reactions to serum.

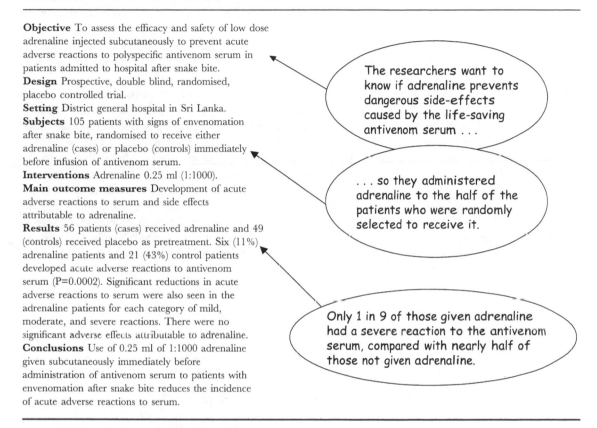

The researchers want to know if adrenaline prevents dangerous side-effects caused by the life-saving antivenom serum . . .

. . . so they administered adrenaline to the half of the patients who were randomly selected to receive it.

Only 1 in 9 of those given adrenaline had a severe reaction to the antivenom serum, compared with nearly half of those not given adrenaline.

FIGURE 6.2 Summary of a randomized controlled trial seeking to identify improvement in care for snake-bite victims

The advantage of these procedures is that the researcher's knowledge of the patient cannot influence the selection procedure. These methods have been proven to reduce selection biases, which otherwise seriously slant the trial results (usually appearing to favour markedly the new or active treatment). Trials that do not adequately report how they concealed allocation of treatment should be treated with suspicion.

This so-called 'concealment of allocation' overlaps with 'blinding' (or 'masking') procedures. Blinding techniques (dealt with in Chapter 13) also involve hiding information about the treatment allocation but are introduced at a later stage in the research investigation where efforts are made to avoid bias in the measurement or experience of outcomes of the treatment under scrutiny.

Consent and Randomization in Trials

Under most circumstances, patients cannot ethically be included in a randomized controlled trial without their informed consent. The information given to patients will usually include both details of the trial and of the nature of randomized allocation of treatment in a trial. However, it is sometimes appropriate to randomize people without their consent, which is sought afterwards. This procedure (shown in Figure 6.3) is sometimes called post-randomization consent or *Zelen's procedure*. Trial participants consent to any treatment and follow-up assessment they receive but without being aware that they have been allocated that treatment by randomization.

The big advantage of randomization is that it deals with confounding so that (provided the trial is big enough to make chance unlikely to affect the result) any differences between patient groups will be due to the treatment offered.

However, there is a catch, since for a variety of reasons many eligible patients do not end up in randomized trials. It may be that clinicians don't like asking their patients, or that, when asked, patients refuse to be randomized. The upshot is that most trials do not study treatments in a fully representative sample of those patients who might be suitable for treatment in the real world.

To put it more technically – randomized controlled trials have high *internal validity* if they are well conducted. That is, their results tell you something real about the effects of treatments because confounding has been dealt with. But they have low *external validity* if only a small proportion of patients agree to participate. That is, you may not be able to generalize the results to the whole group of patients in which you are interested. For this reason it is important to know how many people who were eligible did not participate. Flow diagrams like those recommended by the CONSORT guidelines group can be very useful in identifying the likely impact of non-participation on generalisability.

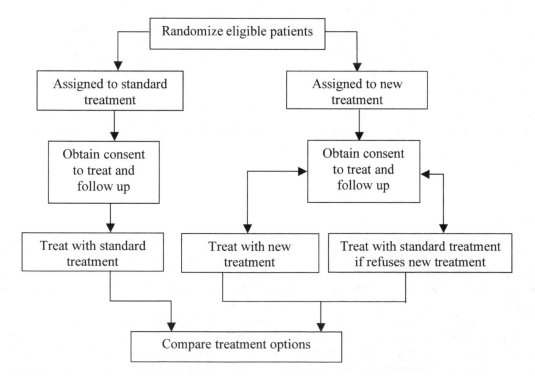

FIGURE 6.3   A flow-chart to illustrate Zelen's procedure for post-randomization consent

PLACEBOS OR TREATMENT-AS-USUAL

We know that when healthcare professionals recommend some course of action, like giving a tablet or encouraging an exercise, it frequently has some beneficial effect – even if the tablet is chalk or the exercise quite unproved in benefit. In a randomized controlled trial in which the people who get the treatment under scrutiny improve more than those who do not get it, it is plausible that the benefit arises only because of this *placebo effect*. To get around such a problem, researchers frequently compare two apparently similar treatments but where only one contains the supposedly active ingredient. Exactly that technique was used by the researchers in the snake-bite study referred to above (Figure 6.4).

Often, it would be unethical to withhold treatment and give placebo, when effective treatments are already available, so a new treatment is tested not against placebo but against one of the standard current treatments. An obvious example arises when comparing two surgical procedures. For example (see Figure 6.5), when they evaluated surgical treatments of heavy menstrual loss, gynaecologists in Aberdeen compared operating time, length of stay in hospital and patient satisfaction in a randomized controlled trial of resection (cutting away) of the uterus lining versus a technique using ablation (destruction) of the lining with microwaves. Plainly, a placebo could not have been an acceptable alternative to the microwave technique. In another case, a new treatment for lowering high blood pressure would usually need to be judged against an existing blood pressure lowering agent; in most circumstances ethics would preclude using placebo when there are available effective treatments.

Low dose subcutaneous adrenaline to prevent acute adverse reactions to antivenom serum in people bitten by snakes: randomised, placebo controlled trial

A P Premawardhena, C E de Silva, M M D Fonseka, S B Gunatilake, H J de Silva

Subjects 105 patients with signs of envenomation after snake bite, randomised to receive either adrenaline (cases) or placebo (controls) immediately before infusion of antivenom serum.

In the snake venom trial, half the patients were given saline, identical in appearance to the adrenaline solution.

FIGURE 6.4 Extract from summary of snake-bite trial (see Figure 6.2) describing the placebo treatment

PRAGMATIC AND EXPLANATORY TRIALS

If a new intervention is to be used in clinical practice then, ideally, its benefits will have been determined in randomized clinical trials. But if these trials have been carried out in narrowly defined ways with carefully selected groups of participants, is it credible that the findings will apply to routine care? Researchers who undertake clinical trials sometimes tackle this challenge – the application of science

Comparison of microwave endometrial ablation and transcervical resection of the endometrium for treatment of heavy menstrual loss: a randomised trial

Kevin G Cooper, Christine Bain, David E Parkin

Background Various new endometrial ablation techniques have emerged for the treatment of menorrhagia. We undertook a randomised controlled trial comparing one new technique, microwave endometrial ablation (MEA), with a proven procedure, transcervical resection of the endometrium (TCRE), for women with heavy menstrual loss.

Methods 263 eligible and consenting women, referred for endometrial ablative surgery, were randomly assigned MEA (Microsulis plc, Waterlooville, Hampshire, UK; n=129) or TCRE (n=134). 230 participants were needed to give 80% power of demonstrating a 15% difference in satisfaction with treatment. All procedures were done under general anaesthesia 5 weeks after endometrial thinning with goserelin 3.6 mg. Questionnaires were completed at recruitment and at 12 months' follow-up. The primary outcome measures were patients' satisfaction with and the acceptability of treatment. Analysis was by intention to treat among women followed up to 12 months (n=116 MEA, n=124 TCRE).

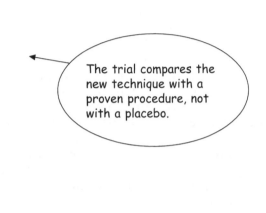

The trial compares the new technique with a proven procedure, not with a placebo.

FIGURE 6.5   Extract from the summary of a randomized controlled trial comparing two procedures to tackle heavy menstrual loss

to the real world – by referring to *explanatory trials* and *pragmatic trials*. An explanatory trial attempts to advance scientific understanding by employing techniques that are like experimental procedures in a laboratory: study subjects are tightly defined with strict inclusion and exclusion criteria, and interventions are similarly narrow – perhaps delivering the same number of milligrammes of a drug per kilogramme of body weight for every participant who has been randomly allocated to the active treatment. A pragmatic trial, on the other hand, is designed with attention to the variability of patients and of their treatments in the routine clinical setting where the treatment is expected to be used.

Put another way, explanatory trials establish benefits that arise in rather idealized conditions, where these benefits are sometimes termed the *efficacy* of the intervention. Pragmatic trials, conversely, offer potentially greater opportunity to generalize the findings, because a range of patients are offered a range of treatments, just as they are in day-to-day practice; this kind of evaluation is sometimes termed the *effectiveness* of the intervention. Figure 6.6 sets out an extract from a pragmatic trial, in which patients with asthma who got a telephone review (the treatment-as-usual control group got a face-to-face consultation with the doctor instead) received a variety of interventions, depending on their responses and what the nurses thought they required. This example demonstrates that, in a pragmatic trial, it is the treatment or management protocol that is under scrutiny, whereas an explanatory trial examines the benefit of a single, highly specific treatment.

Accessibility, acceptability, and effectiveness in primary care of routine telephone review of asthma: pragmatic, randomised controlled trial

Pinnock H, Bawden R, Proctor S, Wolfe S, Scullion J, Price D, Sheikh A

Methods

Recruitment — All four general practices that took part in the study had nurses who were trained and experienced in providing proactive asthma care (table 1). From their computerised asthma registers the practices identified adults (≥ 18 years) who had asked for a bronchodilator inhaler prescription in the previous six months but who had not had a routine asthma review in the preceding 11 months. Patients were excluded if the diagnosis of asthma had been made within the previous year, if they had chronic obstructive pulmonary disease, if communication difficulties made a telephone consultation impossible, or (at the general practitioner's request) for major social or medical reasons. We wrote to all eligible patients inviting them to take part in the study.

Randomisation — Patients were centrally randomised in blocks of 10 to ensure that approximately equal numbers of patients were allocated to each arm of the study.

Intervention — Patients randomised to the telephone review group were sent a letter from their practice informing them that they had been allocated to receive a telephone review and that they should expect a call from the asthma nurse within a month. Nurses were told to make up to four attempts to contact the patient by phone. The nurses were given no instructions about the content of the review except that it should reflect their normal practice and be appropriate to each patient's clinical need. Details about the consultation, including failed attempts at phone calls and the duration of the consultation, were recorded immediately after the review on a piloted consultation record. Nurses arranged any follow up consultations (whether in the surgery or by telephone) they deemed clinically necessary. Patients were free to arrange any consultations they wished.

Control group — Patients randomised to the face to face consultation arm were sent a written invitation to make an appointment to see the asthma nurse within a month. Clinical care and follow up were the same as for the intervention group but without a telephone option.

> There are a few reasonable exclusions but as many patients as possible are included.

> Patients allocated to the telephone review group received variable interventions, depending on their circumstances and the nurse's assessment of need.

FIGURE 6.6 Extract from a pragmatic trial, comparing face-to-face consultation for asthma sufferers with a telephone review by a nurse

INTENTION-TO-TREAT ANALYSIS

The advantages of random allocation to treatments are easily destroyed if some trial subjects are not included in the analysis of the data at the end of the study. For example, some patients do not or cannot take the treatment allocated. If they are excluded from the analysis, the biases removed by the randomization process creep back in. Instead it is recommended practice for all subjects to be analysed within the group they were allocated to – even if they didn't (for whatever reason) experience the treatment. This, at first sight rather odd, principle is known as *intention-to-treat analysis.* The researchers tell us that they used this form of analysis in the gynaecological trial described in Figure 6.5.

To understand the logic of this approach, imagine a trial in which 50 people are randomly allocated to receive Treatment A and 50 people are randomly allocated to receive Treatment B. All 50 people complete their course of Treatment A and at follow-up, half of them have recovered from the condition being treated. In the Treatment B group only one person completes treatment and at follow-up she has recovered. We wouldn't want to argue that Treatment B was better than Treatment A because recovery was 100% for B and only 50% for A; we would want to know what happened to the 49 people who didn't complete Treatment B. Perhaps all of them stopped treatment after a day because of unacceptable side effects, so only 1 in 50 (2%) of patients who took Treatment B actually recovered!

It follows, then, that the intention-to-treat approach can only be fully applied when complete data on the main outcome are available for all participants who were randomly allocated, even if they did not complete the course of treatment. In practice, these outcome data are incomplete in a high proportion of trials. On page 84 we discuss how researchers attempt to deal with the challenge of undertaking an intention-to-treat analysis when they haven't been able to collect follow-up data on all the people who have agreed to participate in a trial.

It is especially important that pragmatic trials, which aim to assess the real-world effectiveness of a treatment, take proper account of everyone who agreed to participate. Sadly though, all the methods proposed (pp. 84–85), for dealing with missing data in trials are less than satisfactory. Consequently, although the assertion of 'intention-to-treat' by a trial's authors is intended to signal a robust analysis, it may simply mask unresolved bias. It is fair to say, however, that a flawed attempt at intention-to-treat is likely to be better than an analysis that pays no attention to participants who underwent random allocation but dropped out somewhere along the way.

To make matters worse, because intention-to-treat analysis has become the customary expectation of those who fund or monitor or publish trials, researchers sometimes use the term loosely – presumably in the hope of impressing those reading their plans or their findings. Surveys of the analyses that are passed off as intention-to-treat show that many of the research studies are poorly described or insufficiently scrupulous in their execution.

III

The Cast: Finding Out About the Subjects of the Research

7

The Research Setting

It can be useful to know where a study is set. As examples of *national studies* there are the confidential inquiries that collect information on all cases of certain types that occur in England and Wales. They include inquiries into perioperative deaths, maternal deaths, and suicides in psychiatric patients (see Figure 7.1).

A *community or population-based study* typically might examine differences between different communities, and look for factors in the environment that might explain such differences. At a more local level it is common to find studies that are *service-based*, for example, in one hospital or clinic or general practice (see Figure 7.2).

The advantages of studies that are based on national data or on large populations are, first, that the results will apply widely, and second that they can examine rare problems, as in the example in Figure 7.3. The disadvantages of national studies are that they are expensive, and it is difficult to collect more than small amounts of information accurately on each case.

The main reasons for doing studies in smaller-scale settings are therefore their lower cost and their ability to collect more information accurately. The main disadvantage is that results may not be generalizable – as, for example, with the description of the neurology practice outlined in Figure 7.2.

Understanding Clinical Papers Second Edition   David Bowers, Allan House, David Owens
© 2006 John Wiley & Sons, Ltd

Suicide within 12 months of contact with mental health services; national clinical survey

Louis Appleby, Jenny Shaw, Tim Amos, Ros McDonnell, Catherine Harris, Kerry McCann, Katy Kiernan, Sue Davies, Harriet Bickley, Rebecca Parsons

Introduction

The national confidential inquiry into suicide and homicide by people with mental illness was established in 1992 and has been based at the University of Manchester since 1996. Its aims are to collect detailed clinical data on people who commit suicide or homicide and who have been in contact with mental health services and to recommend changes to clinical practice and policy that will reduce the risk of suicide and homicide by psychiatric patients.

This national survey is the most recently established of a number of confidential inquiries.

Comprehensive national sample

Information on deaths with a verdict of suicide or an open verdict in a coroner's court was forwarded regularly to the inquiry by the directors of public health in the 105 health authority districts in England and Wales. Open verdicts are often reached in cases of likely suicide and some or all open verdict conventionally included in research on suicide. In this study open verdicts were included unless it was clear that suicide was not considered at inquest – for example, in the cases of children and deaths from unexplained medical causes. These suicides and probable suicides are referred to as suicides in this paper. The sample presented here consists of suicides recorded by directors of public health in the 24 months from 1 April 1996, supplemented with cases recorded as suicide or deaths from undetermined external cause (equivalent to open verdicts) obtained from the Office for National Statistics for the same period.

Data are collected through official channels which are already established.

FIGURE 7.1   A national survey of deaths by suicide

Neurological disease, emotional disorder, and disability: they are related. A study of 300 consecutive new referrals to a neurology outpatient department

Alan J Carson, Brigitte Ringbauer, Lesley MacKenzie, Charles Warlow, Michael Sharpe

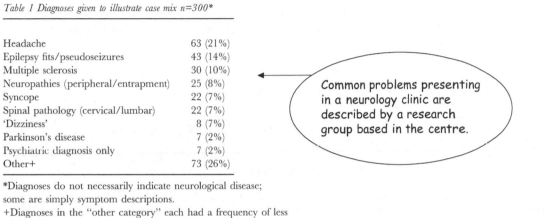

Table 1 Diagnoses given to illustrate case mix n=300*

Headache	63 (21%)
Epilepsy fits/pseudoseizures	43 (14%)
Multiple sclerosis	30 (10%)
Neuropathies (peripheral/entrapment)	25 (8%)
Syncope	22 (7%)
Spinal pathology (cervical/lumbar)	22 (7%)
'Dizziness'	8 (7%)
Parkinson's disease	7 (2%)
Psychiatric diagnosis only	7 (2%)
Other+	73 (26%)

Common problems presenting in a neurology clinic are described by a research group based in the centre.

*Diagnoses do not necessarily indicate neurological disease; some are simply symptom descriptions.
+Diagnoses in the "other category" each had a frequency of less than 2%.

FIGURE 7.2   A study based on consecutive attendances at a clinical service

Sporadic Creutzfeldt-Jakob disease in the United Kingdom: analysis of epidemiological surveillance data for 1970–96

S N Cousens, senior lecturer[a] M Zeidler, research registrar,[b] T F Esmonde, research registrar,[b] R De Silva, research registrar,[b] J W Wilesmith, head of epidemiology department[c] P G Smith, professor of tropical epidemiology and department head,[a] R G Will, consultant neurologist[b]

a Department of Infectious and Tropical Diseases, London School of Hygiene and Tropical Medicine, London WC1E 7HT, b National Creutzfeldt–Jakob Disease Surveillance Unit, Western General Hospital, Edinburgh EH4 2XU, c Central Veterinary Laboratory, Addlestone, Surrey KT15 3NB

Correspondence to: Mr Cousens s.cousens@lshtm.ac.uk

Abstract

Objective: To identify changes in the occurrence of Creutzfeldt-Jakob disease that might be related to the epidemic of bovine spongiform encephalopathy.
Design: Epidemiological surveillance of the United Kingdom population for Creutzfeldt-Jakob disease based on (a) referral of suspected cases by neurologists, neuropathologists, and neurophysiologists and (b) death certificates.
Setting: England and Wales during 1970–84, and whole of the United Kingdom during 1985–96.
Subjects: All 662 patients identified as sporadic cases of Creutzfeldt-Jakob disease.

> Only 662 cases were identified from a population of about 50 million surveyed over more than 25 years.

Main outcome measures: Age distribution of patients, age specific time trends of disease, occupational exposure to cattle, potential exposure to causative agent of bovine spongiform encephalopathy.
Results: During 1970–96 there was an increase in the number of sporadic cases of Creutzfeldt-Jakob disease recorded yearly in England and Wales. The greatest increase was among people aged over 70.

FIGURE 7.3   Data from a unit undertaking surveillance of a rare but important disorder

8

Populations and Samples

Clinical research often involves a study of a group of people, who are taken to represent a wider group to whom the research might apply. The widest group to whom the research might apply is called the *target population*. It might be, for example, 'all insulin-dependent diabetics aged 15–18 years in the United Kingdom'. It would not be feasible to study all the members of such a target population, and it is common therefore to undertake research on a *study population*; for example, 'all insulin-dependent diabetics aged 15–18 years who are recorded on a general practice case-register in six participating practices in West Yorkshire'.

Study populations are often drawn from hospital services. They may not be representative if many sufferers from a disorder do not attend hospital: patients with depression or hypertension, for example. If the majority of sufferers from a disorder do attend a clinic – babies with epilepsy, for example – the study population may still be atypical if the clinic is a specialist or selective one.

SAMPLING

It is very rarely feasible to include all of the study population, so researchers will often take a *sample* from it; for example, 'one in three insulin-dependent diabetics recorded on six general practice case-registers in West Yorkshire'. Sometimes (as in the example in Figure 8.1) a study will use more than one sample.

There are several ways of obtaining a sample from a study population; they are usually called (for obvious reasons) sampling techniques. *Convenience samples* include those whom you encounter and invite to participate, in a haphazard way, for example, by asking colleagues to think of anybody who might be suitable. It is the least satisfactory sampling method, because it may lead to a highly atypical sample but in ways that are not readily identifiable.

Systematic samples include individuals selected on the basis of some regularly occurring and easily identifiable characteristic, for example, first letter of surname; every third patient booked in to see a GP; consecutive attenders on certain weekdays (see Figure 8.2). The problem with this approach is that there may be hidden biases; the people who come to clinic on Mondays may be special in some way which isn't easy to spot.

Random samples avoid these potential biases – at least theoretically; some methods are more random than others! For example, the person undertaking the randomization should be unable to influence the process. Suppose you were taking a 'random' sample of patients on your clinic list; you should not be able to influence the procedure to drop any awkward or aggressive patients who happened to come up in the sample. You must be able to tell what sampling method was used before you can decide whether the sample is representative.

If you want to know whether any conclusions from a research study can be applied in a different setting (that is, how *generalizable* the results are) you must know the relation between each of these – the target population, the study population and the sample.

Understanding Clinical Papers Second Edition   David Bowers, Allan House, David Owens
© 2006 John Wiley & Sons, Ltd

Effectiveness of antismoking telephone helpline: follow up survey

Stephen Platt, Andrew Tannahill, Jonathan Watson,
Elizabeth Fraser

Objective: To evaluate the effectiveness of an antismoking campaign conducted by the Health Education Board for Scotland.
Design: Descriptive survey of adult callers to a telephone helpline (Smokeline) for stopping smoking; panel study of a random sample of adult callers; assessment of prevalence of smoking in Scotland before and after introduction of the helpline.
Setting: Telephone helpline
Subjects: Callers to Smokeline over the initial one-year period. Detailed information was collected on a 10% sample (n=8547). A cohort of adult smokers who called Smokeline (total n=848) was followed up by telephone interview three weeks, six months, and one year after the initial call.
Panel study – Behavioural outcomes were assessed by means of a panel study of adult callers. From the 10% sample of adult callers to Smokeline (see above) a group of 970, of whom 848 (84.4%) were current smokers was randomly selected for follow up at three points in time (three weeks, six months, and 12 months after the initial call). All had consented to participate at the initial interview. Follow up interviews were conducted over the telephone by an independent research team.

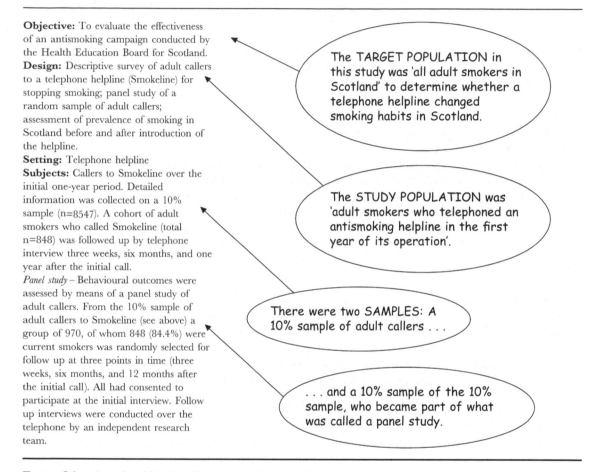

The TARGET POPULATION in this study was 'all adult smokers in Scotland' to determine whether a telephone helpline changed smoking habits in Scotland.

The STUDY POPULATION was 'adult smokers who telephoned an antismoking helpline in the first year of its operation'.

There were two SAMPLES: A 10% sample of adult callers . . .

. . . and a 10% sample of the 10% sample, who became part of what was called a panel study.

FIGURE 8.1   A study which describes two random samples

SAMPLE SIZE AND POWER

One other important characteristic of the sample is its size. However well designed and conducted a piece of research is, it may – if the sample is too small – fail to demonstrate important effects which are truly present in a population (false negative results), or obtain a false positive result by chance (see Figure 8.3).

Researchers should therefore give you one of two pieces of information about their sample. If they were able to choose its size, they should explain how they decided what size to adopt to minimise the possibility of errors, presenting a power calculation which indicates the likelihood that their sample was

A controlled study of fluoxetine and cognitive-behavioural counselling in the treatment of postnatal depression

Louis Appleby, Rachel Warner, Anna Whitton, Brian Faragher

Abstract

Objective: To study the effectiveness of fluoxetine and cognitive-behavioural counselling in depressive illness in postnatal women: to compare fluoxetine and placebo, six sessions and one session of counselling, and combinations of drugs and counselling.

Method

Subjects were women found by screening in an urban health district to be depressed 6–8 weeks after childbirth. From May 1993 to February 1995 women on the maternity wards of two large hospitals in south Manchester were asked to allow assessment of their mood in their homes 6–8 weeks later. This initial approach took place on alternate weekdays; exclusion criteria were inadequate English and living outside the district. The population screened therefore represented a largely unselected systematic sample of newly delivered mothers.

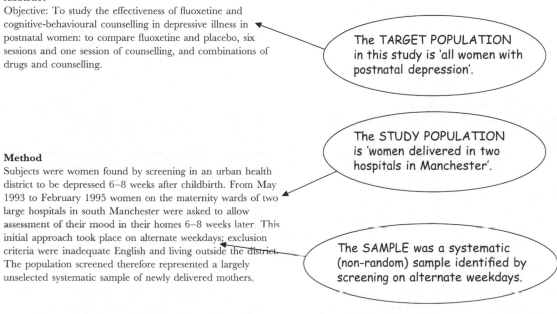

The TARGET POPULATION in this study is 'all women with postnatal depression'.

The STUDY POPULATION is 'women delivered in two hospitals in Manchester'.

The SAMPLE was a systematic (non-random) sample identified by screening on alternate weekdays.

FIGURE 8.2   A systematic sample of patients attending clinics on particular days

large enough to have avoided giving a false negative result. On the other hand, they may not have been able to choose sample size for themselves; perhaps there just weren't funds available or the time or resources to do more than use a sample that presented itself. In this case, researchers should acknowledge their failing and, by the use of confidence intervals, indicate the uncertainty of their findings.

Crisis telephone consultation for deliberate self-harm patients: effects on repetition

M.O. Evans, H.G. Morgan, A. Hayward and D.J. Gunnell

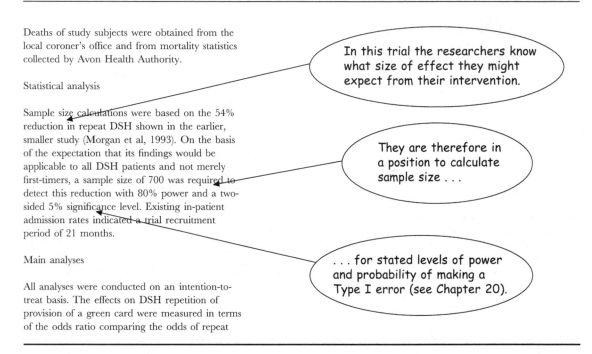

Deaths of study subjects were obtained from the local coroner's office and from mortality statistics collected by Avon Health Authority.

Statistical analysis

Sample size calculations were based on the 54% reduction in repeat DSH shown in the earlier, smaller study (Morgan et al, 1993). On the basis of the expectation that its findings would be applicable to all DSH patients and not merely first-timers, a sample size of 700 was required to detect this reduction with 80% power and a two-sided 5% significance level. Existing in-patient admission rates indicated a trial recruitment period of 21 months.

Main analyses

All analyses were conducted on an intention-to-treat basis. The effects on DSH repetition of provision of a green card were measured in terms of the odds ratio comparing the odds of repeat

In this trial the researchers know what size of effect they might expect from their intervention.

They are therefore in a position to calculate sample size . . .

. . . for stated levels of power and probability of making a Type I error (see Chapter 20).

FIGURE 8.3   Sample size calculation in a clinical trial

9

Identifying and Defining Cases

Once a means of obtaining a sample has been decided, researchers often want to limit the characteristics of individuals included in the sample. They will usually do so by applying inclusion and exclusion criteria.

Inclusion criteria often include an age range, or, for example, the meeting of diagnostic criteria for a particular clinical condition. *Case definition* is aided by the use of standardized criteria. An example includes the International Classification of Diseases (ICD 10). A paper should, where appropriate, always make it clear what criteria were used for case definition.

Exclusion criteria are the other side of the coin. They are the criteria which will lead a subject to be dropped from the study, even though they are in the sample and meet the inclusion criteria. For example, not speaking English may be an exclusion criterion in a psychotherapy trial. Exclusion criteria may lead to a homogenous, clearly defined group of subjects, but one which bears little relation to the real clinical world, so that generalization is difficult. For example, a recent clinical trial of a new drug for the treatment of dementia excluded patients who had any psychiatric history, any neurological disorder, or any other significant physical illness (see Figure 9.1). Since many dementia sufferers have one or other comorbidity, it may not be easy to decide how applicable the trial's results would be in clinical practice.

Once the inclusion and exclusion criteria have been established, they need to be applied to the sample population, to identify and exclude appropriate subjects for the study. For example, it may be that the sample will be screened for a condition, with a more detailed second evaluation for subjects who screened positive. This process may lead to problems if it is inaccurate or biased. For example, if screening involves filling out a questionnaire, then illiterate subjects will not be able to participate unless special arrangements are made.

The final characteristic which determines the nature of subjects in a study is their willingness to participate – that is, to join the study – and their willingness to remain in the study once recruited. *Refusals* are those who decline to participate when they are approached for consent.

Dropouts are those who consent and start the study, but do not complete it. *Losses to follow-up* are those on whom outcome data are not obtained; they are often, but not always, dropouts. If any of these groups is large in relation to the sample it can seriously bias a study, since those who agree to participate in, and complete, a study are not necessarily the same as those who refuse or drop out.

It can be helpful in working out what happened to all the subjects in a study if the authors' account includes a flow chart, as in Figure 9.2.

Understanding Clinical Papers Second Edition   David Bowers, Allan House, David Owens
© 2006 John Wiley & Sons, Ltd

A 24-week, double-blind, placebo-controlled trial of donepezil in patients with Alzheimer's disease

S.L. Rogers, PhD; M.R. Farlow, MD; R.S. Doody, MD, PhD; R. Mohs, PhD; L.T. Friedhoff, MD, PhD; for the Donepezil Study Group

Methods

Patient population. Patients eligible for this study had a diagnosis of uncomplication AD. These men and women of any race aged 50 years or older showed no evidence of insulin-dependent diabetes mellitus or other endocrine disorders; asthma or obstructive pulmonary disease; or clinically significant uncontrolled gastrointestinal, hepatic, or cardiovascular diseases. The diagnosis of probable AD was made according to criteria outlined by the National Institute of Neurological and Communicative Disorders and Alzheimer's Disease and Related Disorders Association (NINCDS-ADRDA), with patients also fitting DSM-III-R illness categories of 290.000 or 290.10, with no clinical or laboratory evidence of a cause other than AD for their dementia. Patients had scores on the Mini-Mental State Examination (MMSE) of 10 to 26, and a Clinical Dementia Rating (CDR) score of 1 (mild dementia) or 2 (moderate dementia) at both screening and baseline. Patients who were known to be hypersensitive to ChE inhibitors or had been taking tacrine and/or other investigational medications within 1 month of baseline were excluded. Concomitant medications such as anticholinergics, anticonvulsants, antidepressants, and antipsychotics were not allowed during the course of this study. Drugs with CNS activity were either prohibited or partially restricted. All other medications were permitted. Patients were required to have a reliable caregiver. Written informed consent was obtained from both the patient and from their caregiver.

Exclusion criteria were relative youth or the presence of other physical illnesses.

Inclusion criteria were based on case definition and scores on measures of intellectual impairment.

Further exclusions were applied to restrict the use of other drugs during the trial . . .

. . . and a further inclusion criterion was the presence of a caregiver.

FIGURE 9.1 Inclusion and exclusion criteria applied to recruits into a trial of a new drug for the treatment of dementia

Effect of consumption of food cooked in iron pots on iron status and growth of young children: a randomised trial

Abdulaziz A Adish, Steven A Esrey, Theresa W Gyorkos, Johanne Jean-Baptiste, Arezoo Rojhani

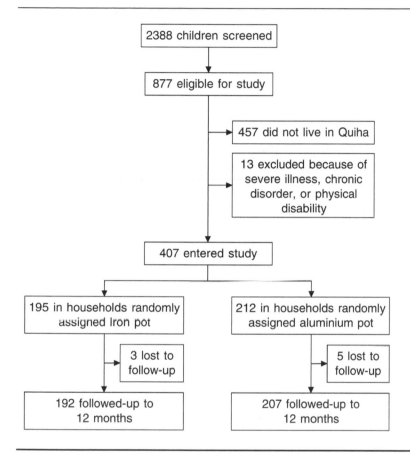

FIGURE 9.2   Flow chart describing the cases included in a randomized controlled trial

10

Controls and Comparisons

Often, results from a particular sample make sense only when they can be compared with those from another. For example, knowing the incidence rate of new-variant CJD in the United Kingdom is interesting in its own right, but it might also be interesting to know the rate in other European countries. People may develop lung cancer even when they don't smoke, but live with somebody who does. But do they develop lung cancer more often than non-smokers who don't live with a smoker?

There are several ways by which authors might obtain comparison data for use in their own study. A common example is the use of 'normal ranges' for tests. This is especially useful when comparison data would be difficult to collect. For example, in the study illustrated in Figure 10.1, the researchers wanted to know if there are national differences in male penis size, since condoms tend to be marketed on a 'one-size-fits-all' basis. This is an important question, because mis-fitting condoms are more likely to split or slip off, but it would not be easy for one group to do all the international work necessary. As it happens, it wasn't necessary.

Sometimes it is common sense to use normal ranges. We can't check the population range of haemoglobin afresh for every study that reports it! On the other hand, published norms may be misleading if they were obtained a long time ago or from a very different population. This became such

Erect penile size of Korean men

Jung Ho Han, Sang Hwa Park, Bon Sam Lee and Sang Un Choi
Institute of Reproductive Medicine

Authors (and country)	Age	n	Total length in mm (SD)[a]	Circumference in mm[b] (SD) Glans	Shaft	Base
This study (Korea)	20–38	279	126.6 (13.4)	113.3 (11.3)	107.5 (10.0)	112.8 (11.4)
Chung (Korea)	20–31	702	127	110.6	–	–
Yoon et al (Korea)	18–25	150	134 (14)	–	112 (11)	–
Park et al (Korea)	20–70	309	118.8 (13.2)	–	121.1 (11.0)	–
Richters et al (Australia)	18–55	156	159.9	119.3	124.0	134.7
Wessells et al (USA)	21–82	80	128.9 (29.1)	–	123.0 (13.1)	–
Jamison & Gebhard (USA)	20–59	2770	157.7 (19.6)	–	123.2 (18.0)	–
Da Ros et al (Brazil)	NA	150	145	110.5	119.2	–
Ng & Tan (Malaysia)	22–70	74	121.1 (17.0)	–	–	–
		11 (Indians)	138.0	–	–	–
		16 (Malays)	123	–	–	–
		46 (Chinese)	116	–	–	–

Notes: *(a)* SD = standard deviation, *(b)* Maximum circumference.

FIGURE 10.1 Use of published norms to compare with newly generated data

a problem with the most widely used IQ testing battery (the Weschler Adult Intelligence Scales, WAIS) that the whole measure was recently redesigned and applied to a new population so that an up-to-date range of reference values could be produced. The Tanner charts widely used to judge children's growth have been revised in the same way. But there are many published results which are not so up-to-date.

A second approach is to use an historical comparison group, so that results produced now are compared with those produced some time previously. The problem with this approach is that it really isn't possible to explain any differences between the 'then and now' groups, because so many things may have changed in the time between the two studies.

The third and commonest approach is therefore to obtain a comparison group from the same population as the sample, and study both at the same time. The comparison group may be identified in a systematic way: For example, suppose the main study is concerned with outcome of hospital admission for myocardial infarction among Asian men, then we might construct a comparison group by taking the next two non-Asian men admitted after each Asian subject included in our study. Alternatively the comparison subjects might be taken entirely at random from the same population as the sample.

One particular type of comparison subject is a *control*, who is somebody who comes from the same population as the subjects, but does *not* have the condition which defines the subjects. That condition might be:

- a disease, such as cancer – as in a case–control study (Chapter 5), where cases and controls come from the same population, but only cases have the disorder of interest;

- exposure to a risk, such as smoking or hypertension – as in an cohort analytic study (Chapter 5), where controls are defined as those who have not been exposed to the risk of interest;

- exposure to a treatment – as in a randomized controlled trial, where the controls receive either no treatment or placebo (Chapter 6).

There is no reason why researchers should restrict themselves to one control group, and in more complex studies they may choose two or more, as in the example shown in Figure 10.2.

Sometimes simply taking a control sample at random isn't enough. For example, suppose a group of researchers wanted to study the health needs of recent immigrants, to find out if they were greater than the local population. Recent immigrants tend to be predominantly young people, while a random sample from the native population would contain all ages. There would be difficulties comparing the health of two groups whose average age was different.

This is a particular example of a common problem known as *confounding*. What happens is that a variable (called a *confounder*) is associated with both exposure and outcome in a study. In this example, age is a confounder – it is associated with being an immigrant and with healthcare needs. Confounders cause problems because they can make it look as if there is a direct association between variables when there isn't really. Alternatively, confounding may mask an association which is really present. For example, if we compared immigrants with the total native population, we might miss a link between ill-health and immigrant status: the immigrants may seem as healthy as the natives but wouldn't be *if we took their age into account* (see also Chapter 24). This sort of *negative confounding* is much less common than confounding which leads to an apparent association between two variables which aren't directly associated.

One way round confounding is to take a random sample and then adjust for the effects of a confounder such as age in the analysis (see Chapters 24 and 25). Another approach is to take a *matched sample* of controls, in which only controls are included who are (say) of the same sex and same age as the subjects.

Controls aren't always randomly selected, as in the example in Figure 10.3.

Finally, check whether the authors have used enough controls, and if they have justified the size of the control group – which is just as important as sample size in the main study group. There's nothing magic about having the same number of controls as cases; in fact, it's often a good idea to have more controls than cases (particularly if the number of cases is small) because it increases the *power* of the study (Chapter 8).

Health of UK servicemen who served in Persian Gulf War

Catherine Unwin, Nick Blatchley, William Coker, Susan Fery, Matthew Hotopf, Lis Hull, Khalida Ismail, Ian Palmer, Anthony David, Simon Wessley

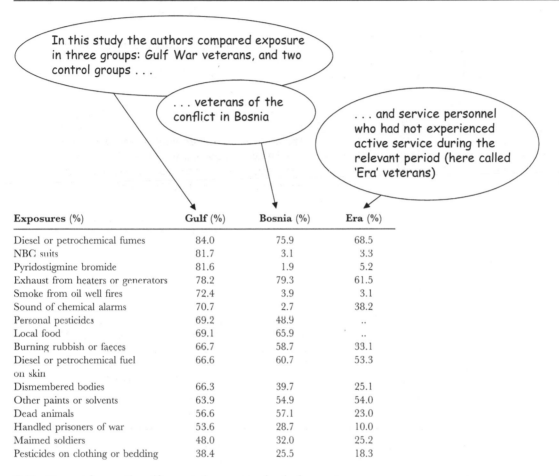

In this study the authors compared exposure in three groups: Gulf War veterans, and two control groups . . .

. . . veterans of the conflict in Bosnia

. . . and service personnel who had not experienced active service during the relevant period (here called 'Era' veterans)

Exposures (%)	Gulf (%)	Bosnia (%)	Era (%)
Diesel or petrochemical fumes	84.0	75.9	68.5
NBC suits	81.7	3.1	3.3
Pyridostigmine bromide	81.6	1.9	5.2
Exhaust from heaters or generators	78.2	79.3	61.5
Smoke from oil well fires	72.4	3.9	3.1
Sound of chemical alarms	70.7	2.7	38.2
Personal pesticides	69.2	48.9	..
Local food	69.1	65.9	..
Burning rubbish or faeces	66.7	58.7	33.1
Diesel or petrochemical fuel on skin	66.6	60.7	53.3
Dismembered bodies	66.3	39.7	25.1
Other paints or solvents	63.9	54.9	54.0
Dead animals	56.6	57.1	23.0
Handled prisoners of war	53.6	28.7	10.0
Maimed soldiers	48.0	32.0	25.2
Pesticides on clothing or bedding	38.4	25.5	18.3

Table: **15 most frequently self-reported exposures by deployment**

FIGURE 10.2   A study using two control groups

Raising research awareness among midwives and nurses: does it work?

V. Hundley, J. Milne, L. Leighton-Beck, W. Graham & A. Fitzmaurice

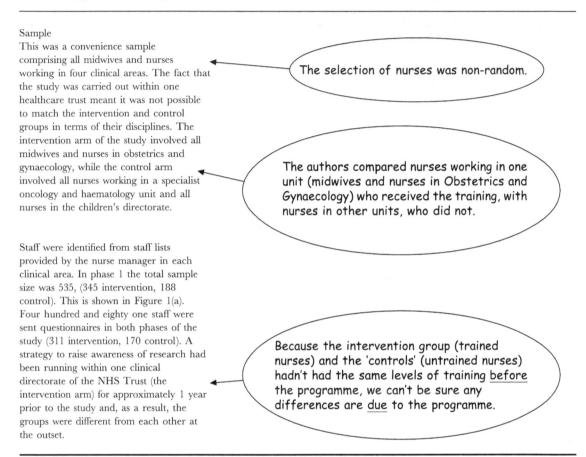

Sample
This was a convenience sample comprising all midwives and nurses working in four clinical areas. The fact that the study was carried out within one healthcare trust meant it was not possible to match the intervention and control groups in terms of their disciplines. The intervention arm of the study involved all midwives and nurses in obstetrics and gynaecology, while the control arm involved all nurses working in a specialist oncology and haematology unit and all nurses in the children's directorate.

Staff were identified from staff lists provided by the nurse manager in each clinical area. In phase 1 the total sample size was 535, (345 intervention, 188 control). This is shown in Figure 1(a). Four hundred and eighty one staff were sent questionnaires in both phases of the study (311 intervention, 170 control). A strategy to raise awareness of research had been running within one clinical directorate of the NHS Trust (the intervention arm) for approximately 1 year prior to the study and, as a result, the groups were different from each other at the outset.

The selection of nurses was non-random.

The authors compared nurses working in one unit (midwives and nurses in Obstetrics and Gynaecology) who received the training, with nurses in other units, who did not.

Because the intervention group (trained nurses) and the 'controls' (untrained nurses) hadn't had the same levels of training before the programme, we can't be sure any differences are due to the programme.

FIGURE 10.3   Non-random selection of intervention and control groups in a trial

IV

Establishing the Facts:
Starting with Basic Observations

11

Identifying the Characteristics of Data

Many of the remaining chapters in this book offer guidance in understanding the various methods that authors use for the presentation and analysis of research data. When you read a few clinical papers which contain any form of statistical analysis, it doesn't take long to realize that authors use a wide variety of procedures, both simple and complex, to analyse data. But whatever procedure they use, their choice will depend, above all, on two considerations, both of which relate to the data in question; that is:

- the *type of data* values involved;
- how these data values are distributed – their *shape*.

By 'shape' we mean: Are most of the values bunched up together in the middle of their possible range? Are they clustered together at the top or bottom of the range? Are they spread out fairly evenly over the whole range? And so on.

When you read a paper it's important to be able to tell the types of data analysed and the shapes of their distributions; only then will you be able to judge whether the statistical procedures the researchers have used are appropriate. As you will see, beginning with Chapter 12, the choice of an appropriate procedure is heavily influenced by data type and shape. We'll start with data type.

TYPES OF VARIABLE – TYPES OF DATA

Variables are things that can change their value, either from person to person, and/or over time. For example, age and blood type are both variables. When we measure a variable we get *data*. There are two broad types of variables, *categorical* variables and *metric* variables. When we measure the value of a categorical variable, we get categorical data; when we measure the value of a metric variable, we get metric data. In this chapter we are going to discuss the characteristics of data in a bit more detail.

Categorical Data

Categorical data has two subtypes:

- *Nominal categorical* (or *nominal*) data can only be *categorized* (assigned into one of a number of discrete categories) but not *measured*. Data on sex, marital status, cause of death, blood type, etc. are nominal. Crucially, the *ordering* of the categories is arbitrary. For example, suppose the blood types of five neonates are AB, B, O, A, and O. These values constitute the categories, which we can be recorded in any order, e.g. as A, AB, B, O or O, B, AB, A, and so on.

Understanding Clinical Papers Second Edition   David Bowers, Allan House, David Owens
© 2006 John Wiley & Sons, Ltd

- *Ordinal categorical* (or *ordinal*) data can be assigned into categories which have a natural *ordering*. For example, suppose the one-minute Apgar[*], scores of the five neonates are measured as 4, 3, 7, 6, 8. These scores constitute the categories, which would be naturally ordered as 3, 4, 6, 7, 8.

Examples of ordinal data are the stages of breast cancer (with naturally ordered categories of Stage I, Stage II, etc.), levels of patient satisfaction (naturally ordered as very unsatisfied, unsatisfied, satisfied, very satisfied), and Glasgow Coma Scale scores (ordered 3, 4, 5,..., 15).

It is important to note that ordinal data are not true numbers. This is because scoring usually depends on judgement and observation (and often on the quality of a patient's response) rather than on proper *measurement*. The consequence is that *the difference between adjacent scores is not necessarily the same*. So the *difference* in health between, say, Apgar scores of 4 and 5 is not necessarily equal to the difference between scores of 5 and 6. Nor is a baby with an Apgar score of 8 necessarily *exactly* twice as healthy as one with a score of 4.

It's this quality of ordinal data which makes some statistical procedures inappropriate. For example, it doesn't make much sense to calculate the average of a set of ordinal scores, if we're not sure of the exact size of the values we're adding up! However, there are appropriate methods for dealing with these sorts of data. We'll start to see how in Chapter 12.

Metric Data

Metric data has two subtypes: continuous data and discrete data.

Continuous Data

Metric continuous data usually result from *measuring* things. The values can lie anywhere within the possible range. Examples are weight (g), serum cholesterol (mmol/1), time on waiting list (weeks), temperature (°C), and so on. In theory, an infinite number of values is possible, although in practice we are usually limited by the accuracy of our measuring device as to what value we actually *record*.

In contrast to categorical data, metric data *are* true numbers. A baby weighing 4000 g is exactly twice as heavy as one of 2000 g, and the difference between babies of 3000 g and 3001 g is exactly the same as that between babies of 4180 g and 4181 g. This means that, unlike with ordinal data, we can legitimately perform arithmetic operations on it. (Note: metric data are also known as *interval-ratio* data.)

Discrete Data

Discrete metric data are invariably whole numbers (*integers*, to be technical) and arise from *counting* things. In contrast to metric continuous data, the number of possible values is limited or finite.

For example, if you are measuring parity (number of previous children) in a group of expectant mothers, possible values are, 0, 1, 2, 3, 4, etc. (values such as 3.6 or 1.5 are not possible). Consequently, the difference between *any* two adjacent values is always exactly the same. So that, in contrast to ordinal data, a parity of 4 is *exactly* twice a parity of 2.

_____

[*]The Apgar Scale is used to assess the well-being of newborn babies. Each baby is scored on five variables (each with possible scores of 0, 1 or 2), i.e. heart rate, respiratory effort, muscle tone, reflex, and skin colour. Total scores can thus vary from 0 (least well) to a maximum of 10. We will have more to say on measurement scales in Chapter 15.

IDENTIFYING DATA TYPE

Figure 11.1 might help you to identify data type (should you need it). One distinguishing feature of metric data is that they almost always have units of measurement attached to them: 10.5 *kg*, 12 *hours*, 1.6 *metres*, 140 *outpatients*, 6 *deaths*, and so on. Categorical data do not. A baby is said to have an Apgar score of just 8, not 8 'Apgars'.

As we've seen, the major division in the world of data is that between categorical data and metric data, sometimes referred to as *qualitative* and *quantitative* data respectively. In the first of the studies below (Figure 11.2), the authors have used a number of different data types to summarize the basic characteristics of the two groups of children used in a trial of the effectiveness of two head-lice lotions. Note that the use of the '+' signs in the evaluation of infestation is not meant to correspond to any *exact* number. These are ordinal measures: '+ + +' is greater than '++', and '++' is greater than '+', and so on. The *number* of live nits could have been recorded as discrete metric data but the difficulty of counting them exactly makes this impractical.

In the next example (Figure 11.3) the authors were comparing the efficacy of integrin β_3 in protecting against myocardial ischaemic events. Their baseline table is shown. Notice in particular that the days since the *previous infarction* data are metric discrete. However, the authors have chosen to aggregate them into four *ordinal* groups. We can say that the time since the last infarction for an individual in the < 8 days group is shorter than the corresponding time for an individual in the 8–30 days group, but we cannot say exactly how much shorter.

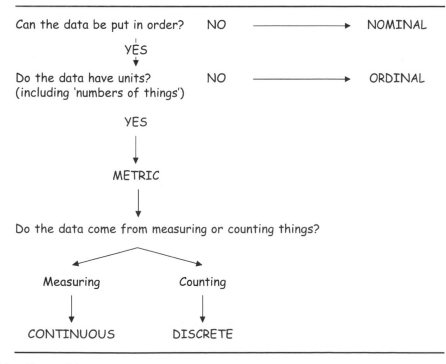

FIGURE 11.1 Types of data

Controlled study of malathion and *d*-phenothrin lotions for *Pediculus humanus* var *capitis*-infested schoolchildren

Olivier Chosidow, Claude Chastang, Caroline Brue, Elisabeth Bouvet, Mohand Izri, Nicole Monteny, Sylvie Bastuji-Garin, Jean-Jacques Rousset, Jean Revuz

Age is metric continuous.		

Characteristic	Malathion (n=95)	*d*-phenothrin (n=98)
Age of randomisation (yr)	8.6 (1.6)	8.9 (1.6)
Sex—no. of children (%)		
Male	31 (33)	41 (42)
Female	64 (67)	57 (58)
Home no (mean)		
Number of rooms	3.3 (1.2)	3.3 (1.8)
Length of hair—no of children (%)*		
Long	37 (39)	20 (21)
Mid-long	23 (24)	33 (34)
Short	35 (37)	44 (45)
Colour of hair—no of children (%)		
Blond	15 (16)	18 (18)
Brown	49 (52)	55 (56)
Red	4 (4)	4 (4)
Dark	27 (28)	21 (22)
Texture of hair—no of children (%)		
Straight	67 (71)	69 (70)
Curly	19 (20)	25 (26)
Frizzy/kinky	9 (9)	4 (4)
Pruritus—no of children (%)	54 (57)	65 (66)
Excoriations—no of children (%)	25 (26)	39 (40)
Evaluation of infestation		
Live lice—no of children (%)		
0	18 (19)	24 (24)
+	45 (47)	35 (36)
++	9 (9)	15 (15)
+++	12 (13)	15 (15)
++++	11 (12)	9 (9)
Viable nits—no of children (%)*		
0	19 (20)	8 (8)
+	32 (34)	41 (45)
++	22 (23)	24 (25)
+++	18 (19)	20 (21)
++++	4 (4)	4 (4)

Annotations (ovals pointing to table):

- *Sex is nominal categorical (ordering of Male/Female is arbitrary).*
- *Hair length is ordinal (ordering of length is not arbitrary).*
- *Both hair colour and texture are nominal categorical (arbitrary ordering).*
- *Level of infestation and number of live lice and viable nits are ordinal (natural ordering).*

The 2 groups were similar at baseline except for a significant difference for the length of hair (p=0.02; chi-square). *One value missing in the *d*-phenothrin group.

Table 2: **Baseline characteristics of the *P humanus capitis*-infested schoolchildren assigned to receive malathion or *d*-phenothrin lotion**

FIGURE 11.2   Types of data used to describe the baseline characteristics of subjects in a nit lotion study

Long-term Protection from Myocardial Ischemic Events in a Randomized Trial of Brief Integrin β₃ Blockade with Percutaneous Coronary Intervention

Eric J. Topol, MD; James J. Ferguson, MD; Harlan F. Weisman, MD; James E. Tcheng, MD; Stephen G. Ellis, MD; Neal S. Kleiman, MD; Russell J. Ivanhoe, MD; Ann L. Wang; David P. Miller, MS; Keaven M. Anderson, PhD; Robert M. Califf, MD; for the EPIC Investigator Group

Age and weight are both metric continuous.

Sex, Risk factors & Vascular disease are all nominal.

Previous infarction (days since) is metric continuous, but here is grouped into four ordinal groups.

Diseased vessels (number of) is metric discrete.

Table 1.—Baseline Characteristics of Patients With Complete Long-term Follow-up*

Characteristics	Placebo (n=662)	Bolus (n=663)	Bolus + Infusion (n=678)
Median age, y	61	60	62
Male	484 (73.1)	477 (72.0)	486 (71.7)
Median weight, kg	84	82	82
Risk factors			
Diabetes	168 (25.4)	156 (23.5)	158 (23.3)
Hypertension	362 (54.7)	368 (55.5)	363 (53.5)
Elevated cholesterol	355 (53.6)	368 (55.5)	352 (51.9)
History of smoking	202 (30.5)	232 (35.0)	209 (30.8)
Vascular disease			
Peripheral	55 (8.3)	56 (8.5)	62 (9.1)
Cerebral	20 (3.0)	25 (3.8)	31 (4.6)
Previous infarction			
None	305 (46.1)	275 (41.5)	282 (41.6)
>30 d	160 (24.2)	179 (27.0)	179 (26.4)
8–30 d	83 (12.5)	81 (12.2)	93 (13.7)
<8 d	185 (28.0)	192 (29.0)	192 (28.3)
Previous coronary procedure			
Angioplasty	164 (24.8)	132 (19.9)	149 (22.0)
Bypass surgery	101 (15.3)	94 (14.2)	110 (16.2)
Diseased vessels			
1	358 (54.2)	343 (51.7)	376 (55.5)
2	192 (29.1)	220 (33.2)	211 (31.1)
3	111 (16.8)	100 (15.1)	91 (13.4)
Coronary procedures			
Balloon angioplasty	584 (88.4)	590 (89.3)	593 (87.9)
Atherectomy	29 (4.4)	26 (3.9)	31 (4.6)
Both	35 (5.3)	37 (5.6)	34 (5.0)

*All values are No. (%) except where otherwise indicated.

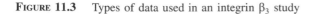

FIGURE 11.3   Types of data used in an integrin β₃ study

SHAPES OF DISTRIBUTIONS

We'll see reasons why the shape of the data distribution is important in a moment, but for now the four distributional shapes most commonly found with clinical data are as follows:

- *Negatively* (or left-) *skewed*. Most of the values lie in the top half of the range, with progressively fewer and fewer values 'tailing' off towards the lower end. (Note that values which lie a considerable distance from the broad mass of values are known as *outliers*.)
- *Positively* (or right-) *skewed*. Most of the values lie in the bottom half of the range, with a longer 'tail' towards the upper end.
- *Uniform*. The values here are spread fairly evenly across the whole range.
- *Mound* or *humped shaped*. Most of the values are clustered around the middle of the range to form a more or less symmetric mound shape, with progressively fewer and fewer values tailing off towards both ends of the range.

We need a particular mention of what is called the *Normal distribution* (dear to the hearts of statisticians everywhere) which is a special case of the symmetric humped distribution. If Normally distributed data are plotted, the result is a smooth symmetric bell-shaped curve, such as that for birthweights in Figure 11.4. When we speak of data being Normally distributed we mean the values form this special bell-like shape. Only metric continuous data can truly be Normal, although the word is widely used to describe any distribution which takes (approximately) this shape. Note that it is good practice always to capitalize the word *Normal* to distinguish it from the word *normal*, used in a more general sense of *usual* or not abnormal.

It is important to know something about distributional shape because a great many statistical procedures depend on the assumptions made about it. For example, some statistical tests should be used only on data which are Normally distributed. These are referred to as *parametric* tests. While other, so-called *distribution-free* or *non-parametric* tests, can be used with any data however distributed. (We'll have more to say on this in Chapter 20.)

The obvious question arises, how can we find out what shape any particular set of data has? In particular, are the data Normally distributed? One way is to draw a *histogram* or *dotplot* of the data (see Chapter 29 for material on charts) and assess the shape visually ('eyeballing'). However, this approach only works if the sample size is large enough (about 100 or more values). Previous experience with similar data may be helpful. There are also analytic methods for measuring Normality, but they are rarely reported. It's also possible to use the value of the standard deviation to do a rough check (although we'll have to leave this until we introduce the idea of standard deviation in Chapter 12). In the absence of any reliable information on distributional shape, authors should play safe, assume a non-Normal distribution, and choose a suitable (non-parametric) statistical procedure. If authors have not done this, then they should provide evidence that they have checked the Normality of the data in question.

A frequency table may also tell you something about the shape of a distribution. For example, in the following study (Figure 11.5), the authors report on the evaluation of a therapy service for adults sexually abused as children. Subjects were interviewed before and after therapy using a number of psychological scales, one of which was the Social Activity and Distress (SAD) scale, which being a scale, produces ordinal data. Although we can often tell quite a lot about the shape of a distribution from a frequency table (as in Figure 11.5), charting it is usually more helpful (and always worthwhile).

In the next example, the authors were investigating the adequacy of hormone replacement therapy for the prevention of osteoporosis. They measured serum E_2 levels in a cross-sectional of 45 patients using transdermal E_2 preparations. Figure 11.6 is the authors' histogram of serum E_2 levels. We can see that

Are clinical criteria just proxies for socioeconomic status? A study of low birth weight in Jamaica

John W Peabody, Paul J Gertler

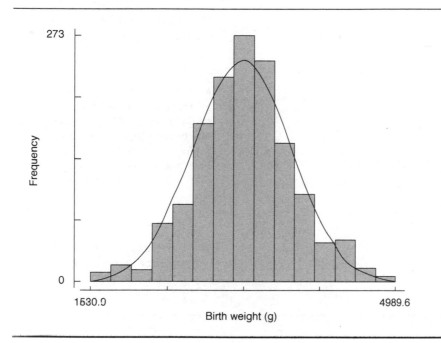

FIGURE 11.4   Normally distributed Jamaican birthweight data

the values tend to cluster in the lower end of the range. The right tail is longer than the left so the distribution is positively skewed. Notice the single high-valued outlier.

Finally, Figure 11.7 shows the distribution of age for a sample of 58 patients in a study of the factors affecting renal failure. This distribution is generally hump-shaped with a small number of low values (or outliers), although we would probably describe it as negatively skewed.

SPOTTING DATA TYPES

To sum up, if data are to be analysed, authors need first to identify the type of data involved, and, second, determine the shape of their distribution. You will not always see references to data type and rarely to evidence on distributional shape in papers.

Even so, as a reader you need to be able to identify what data types are involved (not too difficult now that you know what the possibilities are) if only to satisfy yourself that the most appropriate techniques have been used. If reference is made to either of these aspects of the data, you will probably find them in the Methods/Statistical Analysis section. Here are three brief examples from recent papers:

Adults with a history of child sexual abuse: evaluation of a pilot therapy service

David Smith, Linda Pearce, Mike Pringle, Richard Caplan

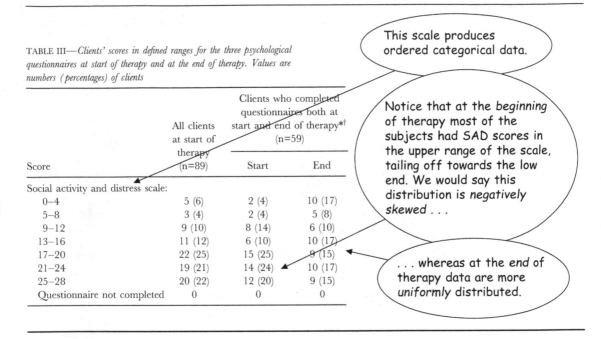

TABLE III—*Clients' scores in defined ranges for the three psychological questionnaires at start of therapy and at the end of therapy. Values are numbers (percentages) of clients*

Score	All clients at start of therapy (n=89)	Clients who completed questionnaires both at start and end of therapy*† (n=59)	
		Start	End
Social activity and distress scale:			
0–4	5 (6)	2 (4)	10 (17)
5–8	3 (4)	2 (4)	5 (8)
9–12	9 (10)	8 (14)	6 (10)
13–16	11 (12)	6 (10)	10 (17)
17–20	22 (25)	15 (25)	9 (15)
21–24	19 (21)	14 (24)	10 (17)
25–28	20 (22)	12 (20)	9 (15)
Questionnaire not completed	0	0	0

This scale produces ordered categorical data.

Notice that at the *beginning* of therapy most of the subjects had SAD scores in the upper range of the scale, tailing off towards the low end. We would say this distribution is *negatively* skewed . . .

. . . whereas at the *end* of therapy data are more *uniformly* distributed.

FIGURE 11.5   Shapes of distributions in abuse study

"Statistical analysis. To compare the fallers and controls we used Student's *t* tests for continuously distributed data, Wilcoxon's non-parametric test for categorical scales (abbreviated mental test score, Barthel index, and transfer and mobility scores), and logistic regression for categorical data. To select variables for construction of the risk assessment tool, we calculated odds ratios for all differences."

"Normally distributed data are summarised by mean (SD) and skewed data by median (inter-quartile range). The Mann–Whitney U test was used to compare continuous data between subgroups. Different episodes in the same child were treated as independent."

"Statistical methods. The distribution of the dependent variable was non-normal: 15% of residents in the survey did not consult a general practitioner, while the distribution for consulters was skewed with a long tail to the right. To allow for this non-normality we conducted a multistage analysis following the approach of Duan and colleagues to examine the demand for medical care under differing types of insurance."

In each of these examples it is clear that the authors' approach is influenced by the type of data and (in the latter two cases) by the Normality or otherwise of the distributions involved.

Adequacy of hormone replacement therapy for osteoporosis prevention assessed by serum oestradiol measurement, and the degree of association with menopausal symptoms

M RODGERS
J E MILLER

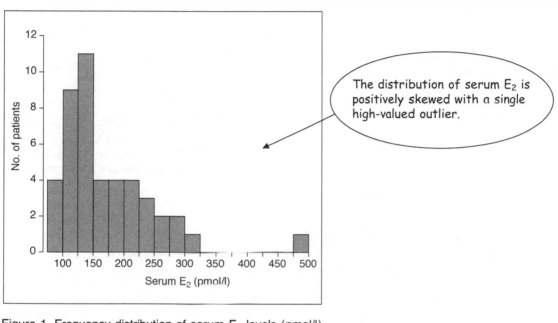

Figure 1. Frequency distribution of serum E_2 levels (pmol/l) in 45 patients on transdermal E_2 preparations.

FIGURE 11.6   Positively skewed distribution of serum E_2 levels, with a single outlier

In this chapter you have seen how important it is for authors to identify data types and distributional shapes if the most appropriate methods of analysis are to be used. So much for the theory. In Chapter 12 you will see some good and bad examples of appropriateness in the analysis of data.

Risk Factors Influencing Survival in Acute Renal Failure Treated by Hemodialysis

John Lien, MD, Victor Chan, MD

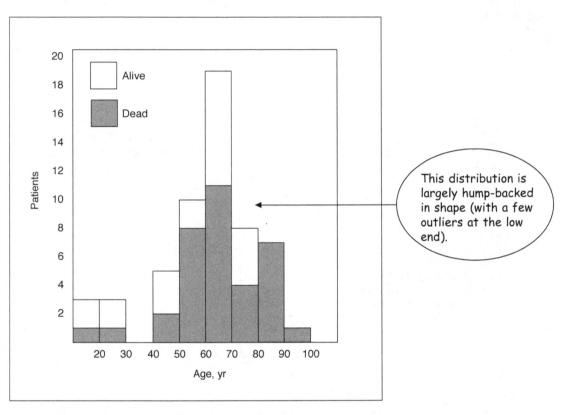

Fig 1.—Histogram depicting mortality (shaded area) in each age group.

FIGURE 11.7   Distribution of mortality in a renal failure study

12

Summarizing the Characteristics of Data

Near the beginning of most quantitative research papers the authors will provide a table which describes the characteristics of the subjects in the study. These *baseline statistics* will usually include *summary measures*, both of the *location* and of the *spread* of the sample data.

A measure of location is the value which best captures or summarizes the point around which the data appear to mass or *locate*. A measure of spread summarizes how much the data are spread out. In this chapter we will see how the choices which authors of clinical papers make between the various summary measures of location and spread are affected by the type of data in question and the shape of their distribution.

SUMMARY MEASURES OF LOCATION

There are two principal measures of location:

- The *mean* (more properly the *arithmetic mean*) is what we all otherwise know as the *average*–simply the sum of the values divided by their number. So we can think of the mean as a summary measure of 'averageness'.
- The *median* is the *middle* value, after all the values have been arranged in ascending order. Thus half of the values will be smaller than the median and half larger. In this sense, the median is a summary measure of 'centralness'.

How is the choice between these two measures affected by data type and distributional shape? Let's start with metric data.

Metric Data

In most circumstances, with a reasonably symmetric distribution, the *mean* is the best measure of location because it uses *all* of the information in the data (and has other advantages). However, if the distribution is markedly *skewed*, the mean will be 'dragged' in the direction of the longer tail by the more extreme values. In these circumstances it might be thought *unrepresentative* of the general mass of the data, and some authors might therefore prefer the median. Because the value of the median depends only on the middle value, it is unaffected by the tail-ends of the distribution, but of course does not use all of the information in the data.

For example, suppose two GPs spent the following consultation times (in minutes) with their last five patients:

Dr A	4, 5, **5**, 5, 6
Dr B	4, 5, **5**, 5, 21

The median (the middle value) is shown in bold. Graphically, we can show these points thus:

Understanding Clinical Papers Second Edition   David Bowers, Allan House, David Owens
© 2006 John Wiley & Sons, Ltd

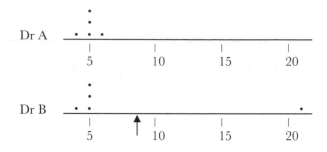

The median and mean consultation times for Dr A are both equal to 5 minutes. For Dr B, the median is still 5 minutes; but with an outlier of 21 minutes, the mean (shown by ↑) increases to 8 minutes. Is 8 minutes really representative of the time spent with the majority of the patients?

Authors might also want to consider the median if the data, though metric, are likely to be *imprecise*, for example, patient self-reporting of their weight or the number of cigarettes they smoked last week. The major disadvantage of the median is that, as we have seen, it ignores most of the information in the data.

So with metric data authors can use *either* measure of location, but their use of the median rather than the mean is an indication either that they particularly want a measure of centralness, they want to compare their results with other results where the median has been used, their data may be skewed, or their data are thought to be imprecise in some way.

Ordinal Data

The most appropriate summary measure for ordinal data, regardless of the shape of the distribution, is the *median*.

We saw in Chapter 11 that ordinal data are not true numbers. As a consequence, the arithmetic operations of addition and division don't make much sense. It follows that authors should not use the mean as a summary measure of location (even with a symmetric distribution), since this involves adding and dividing. In practice, however, old habits die hard and many authors continue to use means. Bear in mind that a lot of data (the severity of any particular injury, for example) form a *continuum* (i.e. from 'no injury' to 'death-causing injury'). We have no way of actually *measuring* such a thing and so use scales which approximate the true underlying values. The more points on the ordinal scale there are, the better the fit is likely to be. If the scale involved contains many values, as, for example, the Apache II scale (a general measure of the severity of a disease, with 72 points), or the Injury Severity Scale (a general measure of the severity of trauma, with 75 points), then the ordinal values might be reasonably close approximations to the underlying true (metric) values. With short scales, like the Apgar or Glasgow Coma scales, equivalence between the values may be poor. In general therefore, if the data are ordinal authors should use the median as the measure of location.

To sum up:

- If the data are metric, authors should use the mean as the most appropriate summary measure of location (unless the data are skewed, in which case they may consider the median as being more representative).
- If the data are ordinal, the median (but *not* the mean) is most appropriate.
- If the data are nominal, no *commonly* used summary measure of location (or spread) is available, but authors will usually summarize their data by describing the proportions or percents of values in each category, for example, stating the percentage of males and females in the sample.

SUMMARY MEASURES OF SPREAD

As well as a summary measure of location, it is usual practice to provide a summary measure of spread, which will capture the degree to which the data are spread out around the mean or median. There are three principal measures available:

- the *standard deviation* (often abbreviated as SD or s.d.)
- the *interquartile range* (sometimes abbreviated as IQR)
- the *range*.

The choice of the most appropriate measure is again influenced by data type and distributional shape. We'll start with metric data.

Metric Data

With metric data, the most appropriate summary measure of spread is the *standard deviation*. Roughly speaking, the standard deviation is a measure of the average distance of the individual data values from their mean. The wider the spread in the data values, the further on average these values will be from the mean, and the larger, therefore, the standard deviation.

For example, consider two more GPs and their consultation times for their last five patients:

$$\text{Dr C} \quad 4, 5, 5, 5, 6$$
$$\text{Dr D} \quad 1, 3, 5, 7, 9$$

We can show this graphically as:

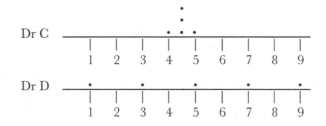

The mean and median consultation times for both doctors are both 5 minutes, but the *spread* of values for Dr D is noticeably wider than for Dr C. The standard deviations reflect this, being 0.707 and 3.160 minutes respectively. So roughly speaking, each of Dr C's consultations is on average only 0.7 minutes from the mean of 5 minutes, while Dr D's are on average more than 3 minutes from the mean of 5 minutes.

The standard deviation is also sensitive to outliers even though the rest of the distribution might be quite narrowly spread. For example, the standard deviations for Drs A and B considered earlier are approximately 0.7 and 7 minutes. Dr B's outlier value of 21 minutes has a dramatic effect on the value of the standard deviation.

Usefully, if the data are *Normally distributed* (or approximately so) then approximately 95 % of the values will lie no further than *two* standard deviations either side of the mean; this may help when you are trying to interpret what a particular standard deviation means. In addition, approximately 99 % of values will lie within *three* standard deviations either side of the mean. We can use this attribute as a rough guide to the Normality or otherwise of the data in question (as we noted in Chapter 11). If we can't fit three standard deviations between the mean and the minimum data value and three between the mean and the maximum value, then the distribution *cannot* be Normal.

On occasion, you may see authors quoting the *range* as a measure of the spread of their data. We discuss the range and its shortcomings in the following section.

With *skewed* metric data, where it has been decided that the median is most appropriate as a measure of location, the interquartile range (see below) is the most appropriate measure of spread.

Ordinal Data

The choice here is between the *range* and the *interquartile range* (IQR). The range is the interval from the smallest value to the largest value. As such, it is much affected by the presence of any outliers. For example, the respective ranges for Drs A and B above are (4 to 6) and (4 to 21) which are quite different. This instability makes the range unsuitable as a measure of spread in most circumstances.

The interquartile range is a measure of the difference between that value *below* which a quarter of the values lie (known as the *first quartile*), and that value *above* which a quarter of the values lie (known as the *third quartile*). The interquartile range is thus a measure of the spread of the *middle 50% of values*.

These ideas are illustrated in Figure 12.1, which shows the quartiles and interquartile range for some hypothetical systolic blood pressure data. Since both ends of the distribution are discarded when the median is determined, so will be any outliers. The interquartile range is thus insensitive to the presence of outliers, and like the median, is a very stable measure.

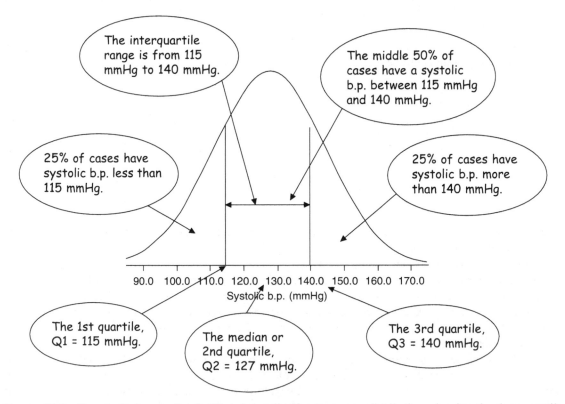

FIGURE 12.1 Hypothetical normally distributed systolic blood pressure distribution, showing the three quartile values and the interquartile range

To sum up:

- If the data are metric, the standard deviation is most appropriate as a summary measure of spread (unless the data are skewed, in which case the interquartile range might be considered).
- If the data are ordinal, the interquartile range (or the *range* if there are no outliers) is most appropriate, *not* the standard deviation.
- The mean should *always* be paired with the standard deviation, the median with the interquartile range or range.

Unfortunately, although a number of summary measures of spread for *nominal* data do exist – see Bowers (1996) for some examples – they have not found common usage and are very rarely seen.

In the study which follows (Figure 12.2) the authors report the results of a study to determine whether a blockade of epidural analgesia (epidural bupivacaine) administered before limb amputation reduced post-amputation pain. One group of patients received the bupivacaine blockade, the other (control) group received saline. The authors' first table describes the baseline characteristics of both groups of patients.

Notice that the authors, having used the mean and standard deviation for age (metric data), preferred to use the median and the interquartile range to summarize daily opioid consumption at admission, which is also metric. As we saw above, this may be because they suspected that the data were skewed and wanted more representative measures than the mean and standard deviation would provide (or they suspected its preciseness, or they particularly wanted a summary measure which captured 'centralness').

Their opioid consumption results show that the median daily level of opioid used at admission in the blockade group (those having the bupivacaine), was 50 mg. This means that half of the group had an opioid consumption less than 50 mg, and half had more. The interquartile range for this group was from 20 mg to 68.8 mg. In other words, a quarter of this group consumed less than 20 mg, a quarter consumed more than 68.8 mg, and the remaining middle 50% used an amount which varied between these two figures. As can be seen, the control group used far less opioids on average, a median of only 30 mg, although the spread in levels of usage was higher (5 to 62.5 mg).

The baseline table will usually contain (as is the case above) more than the summarizing statistics discussed here. We see that information on the proportion of males and females in each group is also given as well as other facts relating to the health of the subjects (whether diabetic, history of previous stroke, previous amputation, etc.) and information on the level of amputation. What information the authors consider relevant and choose to present will depend, of course, on the nature of the study.

In the next study, the authors investigated the exposure to airway irritants in infancy in relation to the later prevalence of bronchial hyper-responsiveness in schoolchildren. They followed two cohorts of infants into childhood, one group (the *Index* group) from a heavily air-polluted town, the second from a town with very little air pollution. Figure 12.3 summarizes the exposure to sulphur dioxide and fluoride by age of the children in the polluted town.

Although the data on pollution concentrations are metric, the authors have used the median (perhaps because of skewness) as their summary measure of average. Instead of the interquartile range, the 10th to the 90th centiles are used as a summary measure of spread (this is akin to the range, but with the bottom 10% and top 10% of ages removed, which makes it more stable). Thus 10% of the children were aged less than the 10th percentile value of age, and 10% were older than the 90th percentile. The infants aged from 0 to 12 months had received an average exposure to sulphur dioxide of 37.1 μ/m^3, 10% of them were exposed to less than 29.5 $\mu g/m^3$, 10% to more than 46.6 $\mu g/m^3$, and 80% had been exposed to sulphur dioxide at levels between these two figures.

In the last of these examples the authors investigated the prognostic factors for recovery from back pain. Their baseline table is shown below (Figure 12.4). They have used the median and range as summary measures for duration of index episode, though the data are metric, possibly because of a

Randomised trial of epidural bupivacaine and morphine in prevention of stump and phantom pain in lower-limb amputation

Lone Nikolajsen, Susanne Ilkjaer, Jørgen H Christensen, Karsten Krøner, Troels S Jensen

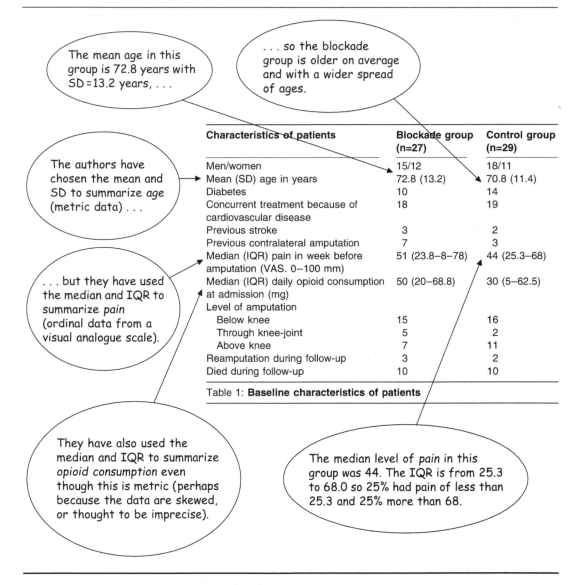

The mean age in this group is 72.8 years with SD = 13.2 years, . . .

. . . so the blockade group is older on average and with a wider spread of ages.

The authors have chosen the mean and SD to summarize *age* (metric data) . . .

. . . but they have used the median and IQR to summarize *pain* (ordinal data from a visual analogue scale).

They have also used the median and IQR to summarize *opioid consumption* even though this is metric (perhaps because the data are skewed, or thought to be imprecise).

The median level of *pain* in this group was 44. The IQR is from 25.3 to 68.0 so 25% had pain of less than 25.3 and 25% more than 68.

Characteristics of patients	Blockade group (n=27)	Control group (n=29)
Men/women	15/12	18/11
Mean (SD) age in years	72.8 (13.2)	70.8 (11.4)
Diabetes	10	14
Concurrent treatment because of cardiovascular disease	18	19
Previous stroke	3	2
Previous contralateral amputation	7	3
Median (IQR) pain in week before amputation (VAS. 0–100 mm)	51 (23.8–8–78)	44 (25.3–68)
Median (IQR) daily opioid consumption at admission (mg)	50 (20–68.8)	30 (5–62.5)
Level of amputation		
Below knee	15	16
Through knee-joint	5	2
Above knee	7	11
Reamputation during follow-up	3	2
Died during follow-up	10	10

Table 1: **Baseline characteristics of patients**

FIGURE 12.2   Baseline characteristics in a post-operative stump pain study

skewed distribution, or perhaps because they believed the patient-recall of episode duration was likely to be imprecise and preferred to treat it as if it would yield ordinal data.

They have *inappropriately* used the mean and standard deviation as summary measures for the pain scores and the disability questionnaire scores, both of which are ordinal with short scales (see Chapter 11). More appropriate would have been the median and the interquartile range.

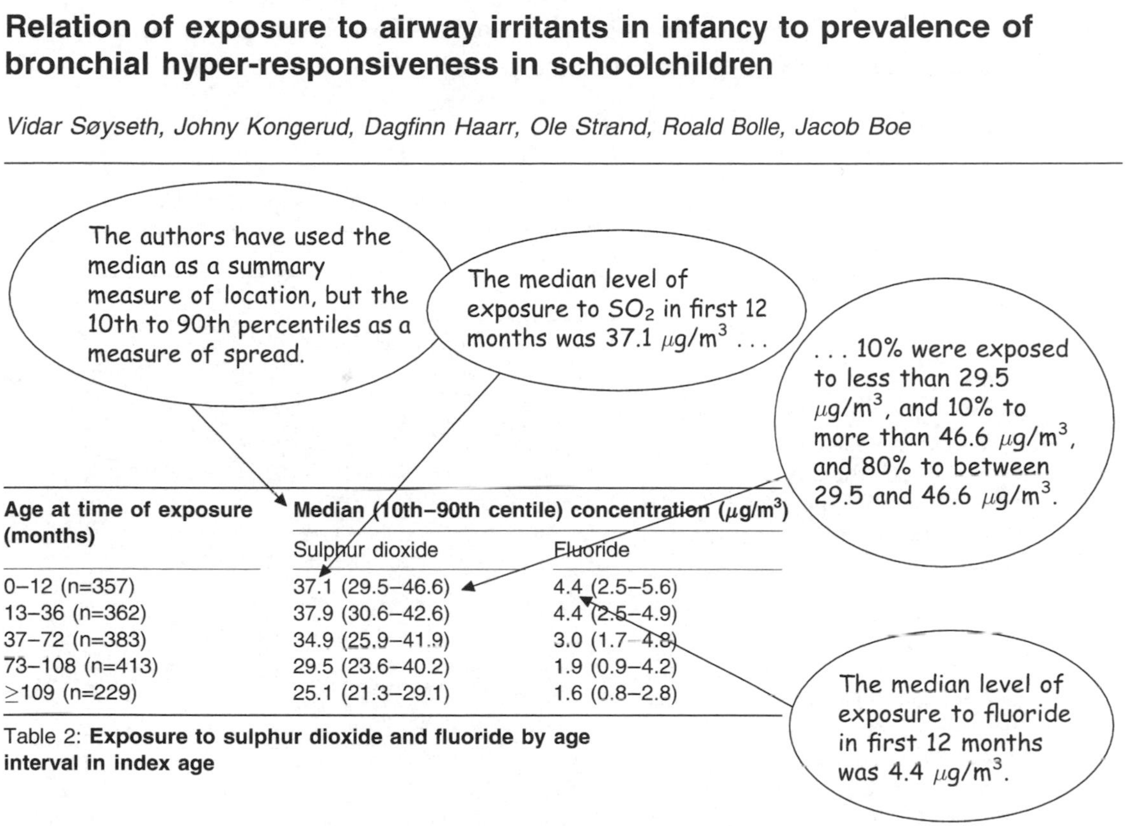

Relation of exposure to airway irritants in infancy to prevalence of bronchial hyper-responsiveness in schoolchildren

Vidar Søyseth, Johny Kongerud, Dagfinn Haarr, Ole Strand, Roald Bolle, Jacob Boe

Age at time of exposure (months)	Median (10th–90th centile) concentration (μg/m^3)	
	Sulphur dioxide	Fluoride
0–12 (n=357)	37.1 (29.5–46.6)	4.4 (2.5–5.6)
13–36 (n=362)	37.9 (30.6–42.6)	4.4 (2.5–4.9)
37–72 (n=383)	34.9 (25.9–41.9)	3.0 (1.7–4.8)
73–108 (n=413)	29.5 (23.6–40.2)	1.9 (0.9–4.2)
≥109 (n=229)	25.1 (21.3–29.1)	1.6 (0.8–2.8)

Table 2: **Exposure to sulphur dioxide and fluoride by age interval in index age**

The authors have used the median as a summary measure of location, but the 10th to 90th percentiles as a measure of spread.
The median level of exposure to SO2 in first 12 months was 37.1 μg/m3 . . .
. . . 10% were exposed to less than 29.5 μg/m3, and 10% to more than 46.6 μg/m3, and 80% to between 29.5 and 46.6 μg/m3.
The median level of exposure to fluoride in first 12 months was 4.4 μg/m3.

FIGURE 12.3 The median and the 10th to 90th centiles used as summary measures of location and spread respectively in the bronchial hyper-responsiveness study

When you read a clinical paper you should be able to tell what summary measures of location and spread the authors have used, and whether their choice is the most appropriate for the types of data involved and their distributional shapes.

The choice of suitable *summary* measures for sample data is not the only decision influenced by the type of data and their distributional shape. As we will see in later chapters, these two factors also have a crucial role in making appropriate choices in many other areas of statistical analysis. Hypothesis testing, which we will consider in Chapter 21, is just one example.

Clinical course and prognostic factors in acute low back pain: an inception cohort study in primary care practice

J Coste, G Delecoeuillerie, A Cohen de Lara, J M Le Parc, J B Paolaggi

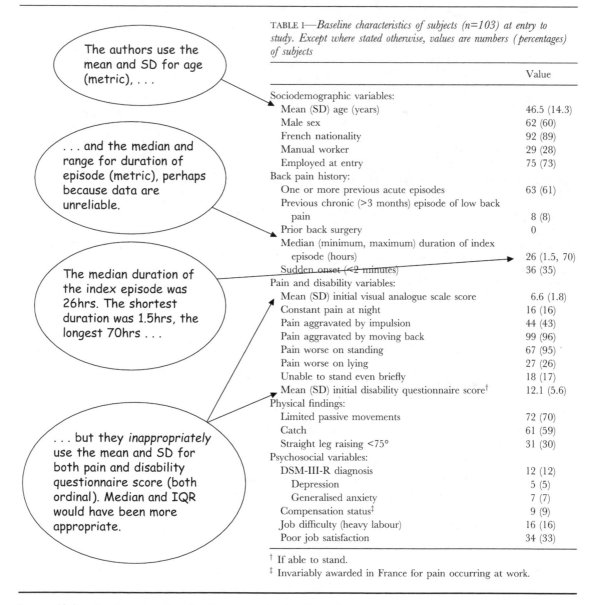

The authors use the mean and SD for age (metric), . . .

. . . and the median and range for duration of episode (metric), perhaps because data are unreliable.

The median duration of the index episode was 26hrs. The shortest duration was 1.5hrs, the longest 70hrs . . .

. . . but they *inappropriately* use the mean and SD for both pain and disability questionnaire score (both ordinal). Median and IQR would have been more appropriate.

TABLE I—*Baseline characteristics of subjects (n=103) at entry to study. Except where stated otherwise, values are numbers (percentages) of subjects*

	Value
Sociodemographic variables:	
Mean (SD) age (years)	46.5 (14.3)
Male sex	62 (60)
French nationality	92 (89)
Manual worker	29 (28)
Employed at entry	75 (73)
Back pain history:	
One or more previous acute episodes	63 (61)
Previous chronic (>3 months) episode of low back pain	8 (8)
Prior back surgery	0
Median (minimum, maximum) duration of index episode (hours)	26 (1.5, 70)
Sudden onset (<2 minutes)	36 (35)
Pain and disability variables:	
Mean (SD) initial visual analogue scale score	6.6 (1.8)
Constant pain at night	16 (16)
Pain aggravated by impulsion	44 (43)
Pain aggravated by moving back	99 (96)
Pain worse on standing	67 (95)
Pain worse on lying	27 (26)
Unable to stand even briefly	18 (17)
Mean (SD) initial disability questionnaire score†	12.1 (5.6)
Physical findings:	
Limited passive movements	72 (70)
Catch	61 (59)
Straight leg raising <75°	31 (30)
Psychosocial variables:	
DSM-III-R diagnosis	12 (12)
Depression	5 (5)
Generalised anxiety	7 (7)
Compensation status‡	9 (9)
Job difficulty (heavy labour)	16 (16)
Poor job satisfaction	34 (33)

† If able to stand.

‡ Invariably awarded in France for pain occurring at work.

FIGURE 12.4   Baseline characteristics in an acute back pain study

13

Measuring the Characteristics of Subjects

Chapter 9 dealt with the issue of inclusion and exclusion criteria for study subjects – who is in and who is out. Once you have worked out how the sample has been assembled according to these criteria, you need to know about their characteristics, so as to judge how close the study subjects are to the patients or clients in your practice. If the study sets out to draw comparisons between two or more groups you will want to know whether the groups are sufficiently comparable.

The extracts in Figure 13.1, from a clinical trial examining one form of social care (called 'case-management') in long-term and severe mental illness, provide a fairly typical illustration of this two-stage research process.

Social services case-management for long-term mental disorders: a randomised controlled trial

M Marshall, A Lockwood, D Gath

Subjects were considered for inclusion if they were judged by the referrer to have a severe, persistent, psychiatric disorder; were homeless (roofless, or living in a night shelter or hostel for the homeless); at risk of homelessness (ie, facing a threat of eviction, or having a recent history of homelessness, or frequent changes of accommodation), living in accommodation which was temporary, or supported (such as a group home), or of poor quality; were coping badly, experiencing social isolation, or causing disturbances; and were not clients of another case-management service.

Subjects who had a well-documented psychiatric history were assessed either by a trained research nurse or a research psychiatrist; others were assessed by a research psychiatrist. One of the authors (MM) then allocated an ICD 10 diagnosis.

Social behaviour was measured by observer ratings and subjects' own ratings. The observer rating of social behaviour was made with a standardised behaviour scale (REHAB), which rates the frequency of items of embarrassing or disruptive behaviour, such as violence, self harm, shouting and swearing, and sexual offensiveness (deviant behaviour); and lack of general skills (general behaviour).[17] REHAB ratings were made by an observer trained by the researchers (eg, a member of staff in a hostel, a voluntary worker, or a primary-care worker). The subject's perception of his or her own social behaviour was rated with the Social Integration Questionnaire.[18] Severity of psychiatric symptoms was assessed with the Manchester Scale.[19]

This section sets out the kind of people the researchers wanted in the study—mainly inclusions with one exclusion.

This section describes how the researchers tried to describe the study subjects and quantify some of their needs, quality of life, and abnormalities of social behaviour.

FIGURE 13.1 Extracts from a clinical trial, describing inclusions, exclusions and some of the baseline measures

Understanding Clinical Papers Second Edition David Bowers, Allan House, David Owens
© 2006 John Wiley & Sons, Ltd

These measures are sometimes called *baseline* measures because they are taken at the start of the study, or *casemix* measures because they describe the mix of cases in the study. You need them not only to check the relevance of the study to your patients or clients, but also, if it is a follow-up study, as a baseline which can be used later to see how much, if at all, they have improved or deteriorated.

In many papers these initial findings are set out in the first table of the results section – showing us the consequences of the inclusion and exclusion process and of sampling. The table shown in Figure 13.2 comes from the 'case management' trial illustrated above.

Social services case-management for long-term mental disorders: a randomised controlled trial

M Marshall, A Lockwood, D Gath

	Control group (n=40)		Case-management (n=40)	
	No	%	No	%
Age grouping				
20–29	4	10.0	4	10.0
30–39	6	15.4	11	28.2
40–49	16	40.0	6	15.4
50–59	5	12.5	9	22.5
60+	9	22.5	9	22.5
Sex				
Male	34	85.0	34	85.0
Female	6	15.0	6	15.0
History				
Illness >1 year	40	100	40	100
Previous psychiatric admission	34	85.0	34	85.0
In contact with psychiatric services	25	62.5	21	52.5
ICD 10 diagnosis				
Schizophrenia and related disorders	32	80.0	27	67.5
Mood disorders	3	7.5	6	15.0
Personality disorder	2	5.0	3	7.5
Neurotic disorders	1	2.5	3	7.5
Organic disorders	2	5.0	1	2.5
Housing status				
Hostels for the homeless	18	45.0	20	50.0
Staffed group homes	7	17.5	4	10.0
Unstaffed group home	5	12.5	5	12.5
Night shelter or sleeping rough	4	10.0	3	7.5
Supported flat	3	7.5	3	7.5
Own flat	2	5.0	3	7.5
Poor quality bedsit	0	0.0	2	5.0
With family	1	2.5	0	0.0

In the case of this trial comparing two treatments, the table needs to show how similar or different the two groups were before the study interventions began.

As it turns out, there are differences, for example, a greater proportion of the case-management group have mood disorders or neurosis and fewer of them are in contact with psychiatric services.

Table 1: **Characteristics of subjects**

FIGURE 13.2 Baseline or casemix measures from a clinical trial

INFORMATION AND MEASUREMENT BIAS

Many assessments – like those in the case-management study – allow for some subjective judgement by the researcher who is trying to rate subjects. Consequently, the researcher's own attitudes (rather than just the characteristics of the subjects) could sway his or her judgement.

This sort of bias is especially likely when researchers are undertaking follow-up assessments in cohort studies or clinical trials. After all, many researchers undertake their investigations because they reckon that a new intervention is a winner, or a particular exposure is a cause of disease. Picture yourself rating outcome; how could you prevent your prior opinions about the treatment, or exposure to some risk, from influencing your measurements?

Study subjects too are influenced by knowing whether they received active or placebo treatment, or old versus new interventions, or whether a study is designed to show a link between a certain exposure and an outcome. First, knowledge about the treatment or exposure will often affect subjects' *judgements* about their symptoms or their experience of disability. Second, the same knowledge can have impact upon their *expression* or *description* of symptoms or disability when they are being rated.

For this reason, researchers often take steps to conceal from the person doing the rating which group the subject has been allocated to or drawn from. This process is referred to as *blinding* or *masking* the rater. In clinical trials, the subject can easily reveal which treatment they received to a rater who is supposed to be blinded to treatment status. For these reasons, attempts are routinely made to blind subjects as well as raters whenever feasible. This process of blinding researcher and subject is referred to as a *double-blind* procedure, *single-blind* referring to situations where one party is aware (usually the subject) but the other is not.

It can be relatively easy to double-blind some drug treatment studies, especially where the manufacturer assists the research by producing and supplying placebo or alternative drugs with identical appearance. Even so, different side-effect profiles mean that clinically aware raters can (or think that they can) readily determine which subjects had which treatments. Many psychological therapies and surgical procedures are not amenable to double-blind techniques. Nevertheless, researchers such as those in the example in Figure 13.3 go to great lengths to achieve as much blinding as possible in rigorous efforts to reduce measurement biases.

In cohort or case–control studies, where the two groups of subjects are not allocated to interventions, the blinding technique is applicable but not always possible. Sometimes researchers make remarkably strenuous efforts to achieve blinding of raters: occasionally going to such lengths as to transcribe interviews so as to remove any visual or verbal clues as to which group the subject belonged and arranging for the rating of these transcripts.

Those asked to extract information from case notes or other routine records may also, on occasions, be blinded to whether the record belongs to a member of the case group or the control group (in a case–control study) or in the group exposed or unexposed to the risk factor (in a cohort analytic study); one such situation is shown in Figure 13.4. The reason for this is that evidence about research biases has shown that the distortions that may result from unblinded studies can be large enough to bring about false findings, either exaggerating or wrongly minimizing the true study results.

BIAS ARISING FROM MISSING VALUES

However careful researchers are, it is all-but-inevitable that there will be missing values in their data. It may be that subjects fail to complete a particular questionnaire, for example, or decline to answer certain questions. In studies which involve some follow-up, there is the additional problem that not all of the original sample may be available for subsequent assessments. This can lead to biased results, if the

Electroconvulsive therapy: results in depressive illness from the Leicestershire trial

S BRANDON, P COWLEY, C McDONALD, P NEVILLE, R PALMER, S WELLSTOOD-EASON

After the initial assessment each patient was allocated a code number and regardless of diagnosis allocated according to previously determined random numbers to receive treatment or placebo (simulated treatment). Elaborate arrangements ensured that research and nursing staff had no opportunity to discover which group the patients were in. Treatment was carried out in "sealed off" electroconvulsive therapy units and administered by a member of the research team who had no access to any other information on the patient. Nurses and anaesthetists had no contact with the patients outside the electroconvulsive therapy suite and were "sworn to secrecy." Other nursing staff had no access to patients during or after treatment until the patient was able to enter the recovery room. We could find no evidence of any breach of security.

In the treatment room all patients received a standard anaesthetic of methohexitone and suxamethonium at a dosage related to body weight (1 mg methohexitone/kg, 0.5 mg suxamethonium/kg). No atropine was used, and oxygenation was maintained throughout. An Ectron Mark IV electroconvulsive therapy machine was used with bilateral temporal

> Even patients who did not receive ECT were anaesthetized, and the treatment suite was closed to all but research staff sworn to secrecy.

FIGURE 13.3 Blinding patients and staff so that measures made later can be masked as to the allocation of subjects to treatment groups

---

missing values are not randomly distributed. That is, if certain subjects (say, women, or the elderly, or people with alcohol dependence, or people assigned to treatment A rather than treatment B) are less likely to complete the measures than others, then the results of the study may be systematically distorted by the absence of results from those subjects. What can the researchers do?

First, they could simply give you data for those measures (or those subjects) on whom it is available. This can be a little confusing if the numbers keep changing, but at least it can help you 'track' the data collection process in the study. Second, researchers can *impute* results for the missing values or subjects. They might do this, for example, by assuming that a missing value was the same as the average for that value in the sample.

Particularly in relation to follow-up studies, researchers have a third option. Suppose they are conducting a study in which assessments are made at baseline and at 3-monthly intervals for a year, so there should be results available for each subject at 0, 3, 6, 9 and 12 months. For obvious reasons, it is the values at later follow-ups that are more likely to be missing. The researchers can decide to assume that each missing value is the same as the last one actually obtained for that subject – the so-called *last observation carried forward* (see Figure 13.5). So if a subject misses (say) her 9- and 12-month follow-up assessments, then the missing values are assumed to be the same as those which *were* obtained at the 6-month assessment.

Missing values in a randomized controlled trial present particular problems. Researchers may simply present results for those subjects on whom they have all assessments, but we know these *trial completers* are not the same as all subjects (they tend to do better than trial dropouts). An alternative is to provide results for all *trial entrants* with missing values for the dropouts imputed. This is known as *intention-to-treat analysis*

Prenatal ultrasound examinations and risk of childhood leukaemia: case-control study

Estelle Naumburg, Rino Bellocco, Sven Cnattingius, Per Hall, Anders Ekbom.

Concerns over a possible association between exposure to ultrasound in utero and an increased risk of childhood malignancies have not been substantiated, but previous studies have been hampered by low statistical power or based on interviews with the parents done retrospectively, or both. To assess the impact of ultrasound and the risks of childhood lymphatic and myeloid leukaemia, we performed a nationwide population based case-control study using prospectively assembled data on prenatal exposure to ultrasound.

Subjects, methods, and results

The cases in this study comprised all children born and diagnosed as having leukaemia between 1973 and 1989 and reported to the nationwide Swedish registers of birth, cancer, and causes of death – in all, 752 cases. One control was randomly selected for each child with leukaemia from the Swedish Birth Registry and matched by sex and year and month of birth. The study was restricted to cases and controls without Down's syndrome (n=731), and medical records of 652 (89%) matched case-control pairs could be retrieved (578 cases with lymphatic leukaemia and 74 with myeloid leukaemia).

Altogether, 361 (48%) of the children with leukaemia had developed it before the age of 4, and 21 children were born in twin pregnancies. Information on exposure was extracted from antenatal, obstetric, and other standardised medical records by one of us (EN), who was blind to whether the child was a case or control. Conditional logistic regression was performed to study the association between prenatal exposure to ultrasound and childhood leukaemia (lymphatic and myeloid leukaemia). Maximum likelihood methods were used to estimate the odds ratio and 95% confidence intervals.

Blinding is about masking group membership from people carrying out any kind of measurement; casenote information is a common target of blinding procedures – for all the same reasons as in direct rating of live participants.

FIGURE 13.4 Blinding people who are extracting casenote information to the participants' group membership (cases or controls)

(see Chapter 6). In Figure 13.5, which comes from a clinical trial evaluating a new anti-dementia drug, the authors explain how they have dealt with missing values at follow-up.

Whichever approach researchers take, you should be able to find an estimate of the possible impact on their results. In other words, they should tell you what effect missing values might have had, and how their results might have been different, if either (a) there were no missing values or (b) they had made different assumptions when imputing the missing values. This sort of calculation is often called a *sensitivity analysis*.

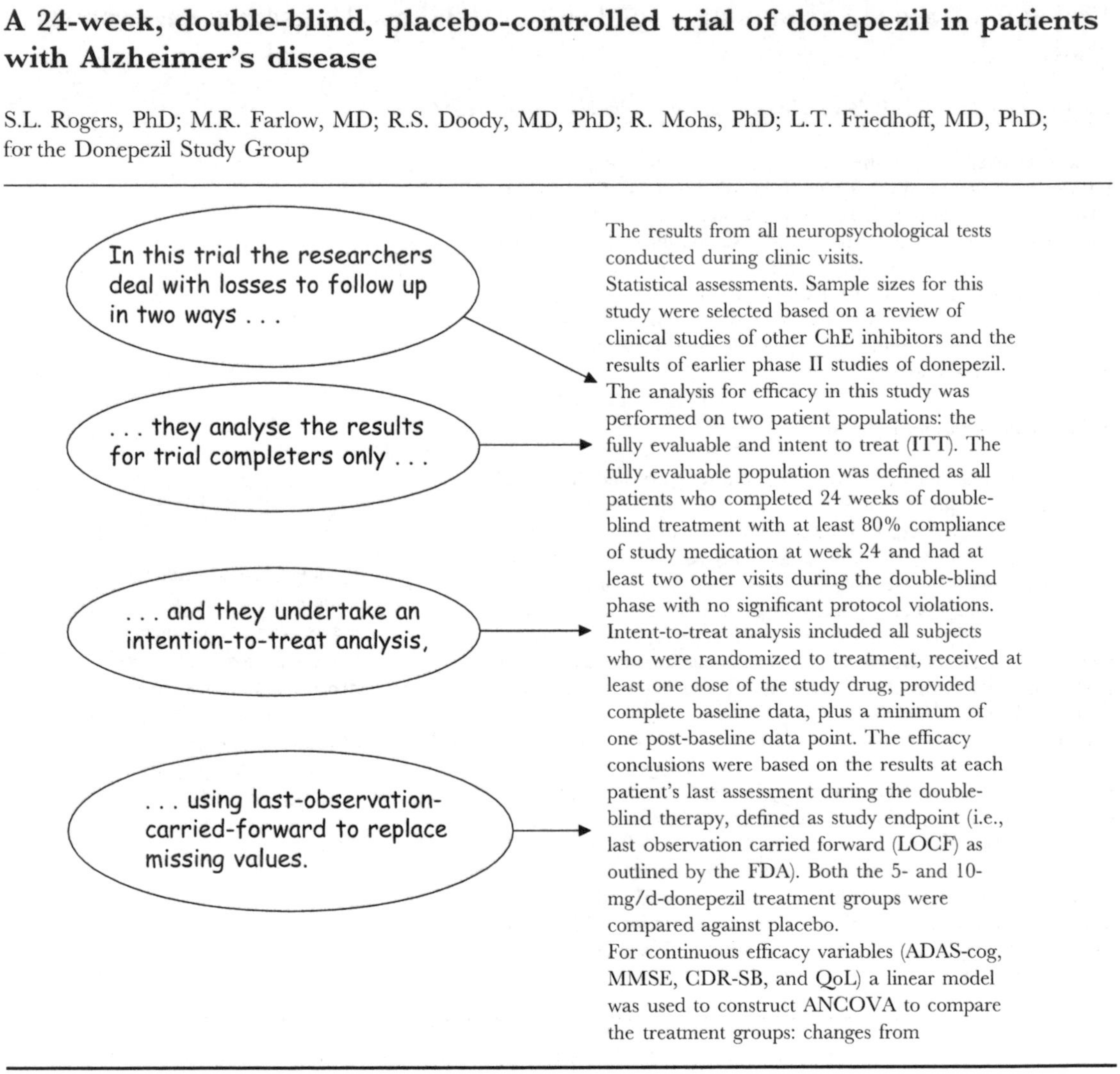

A 24-week, double-blind, placebo-controlled trial of donepezil in patients with Alzheimer's disease

S.L. Rogers, PhD; M.R. Farlow, MD; R.S. Doody, MD, PhD; R. Mohs, PhD; L.T. Friedhoff, MD, PhD; for the Donepezil Study Group

In this trial the researchers deal with losses to follow up in two ways . . .

. . . they analyse the results for trial completers only . . .

. . . and they undertake an intention-to-treat analysis,

. . . using last-observation-carried-forward to replace missing values.

The results from all neuropsychological tests conducted during clinic visits.
Statistical assessments. Sample sizes for this study were selected based on a review of clinical studies of other ChE inhibitors and the results of earlier phase II studies of donepezil. The analysis for efficacy in this study was performed on two patient populations: the fully evaluable and intent to treat (ITT). The fully evaluable population was defined as all patients who completed 24 weeks of double-blind treatment with at least 80% compliance of study medication at week 24 and had at least two other visits during the double-blind phase with no significant protocol violations. Intent-to-treat analysis included all subjects who were randomized to treatment, received at least one dose of the study drug, provided complete baseline data, plus a minimum of one post-baseline data point. The efficacy conclusions were based on the results at each patient's last assessment during the double-blind therapy, defined as study endpoint (i.e., last observation carried forward (LOCF) as outlined by the FDA). Both the 5- and 10-mg/d-donepezil treatment groups were compared against placebo.
For continuous efficacy variables (ADAS-cog, MMSE, CDR-SB, and QoL) a linear model was used to construct ANCOVA to compare the treatment groups: changes from

FIGURE 13.5   Dealing with missing values in a clinical trial

14

Measuring the Characteristics of Measures

You may often see clinical papers containing the results of studies which compare two or more diagnostic tests. More often than not, these studies will compare the performance of a new or improved procedure with a 'gold standard' test, which is assumed to give the correct result – in diagnosis or predicting outcomes for example. We need to say a few words about the ideas which underlie these studies, before we examine some examples from the literature, and point out what you as a reader need to look out for.

Look at Figure 14.1, which shows serum CK-BB concentrations in 70 patients admitted to A & E with typical chest pain suggestive of acute myocardial infarction (AMI). These data are metric continuous. The clinicians involved did not initially know which patients had had an infarction and which not, although in fact 50 had and 20 had not. Action needs to be taken if the patient really has experienced infarction, but not otherwise, and we could use serum CK-BB concentration as our *diagnostic test*, provided we can arrive at an appropriate critical (or cut-off) value with which to inform our decision.

If the physicians involved use a serum CK-BB level of 12 µg/1 as the cut-off, two patients with an infarction will be missed, but no patients will be included who have not had an infarction. If a lower value is used, say 6 µg/1, then all of the patients with an infarction will be detected, but so will 10 (or so) healthy patients. Clearly there is an optimum (but never perfect) cut-off value.

Researchers generally use four separate but interconnected measures of a test's accuracy:

- *sensitivity*: the proportion (or %) of those patients *with* the condition whom the test correctly identifies as having it
- *specificity*: the proportion (or %) of those patients *without* the condition whom the test correctly identifies as not having it
- *positive predictive value* (*PPV*): the proportion (or %) of patients whom the test identifies as having the condition who do have it
- *negative predictive value* (*NPV*): the proportion (or %) of patients whom the test does not identify as having the condition who do not have it.

Clearly, the predictive diagnostics, positive and negative predictive values, are clinically more useful. As a clinician you want to know, for example, the chances of a patient having the condition if they return a positive test result (positive predictive value), rather than whether they will give a positive test result if they are known to have the condition (sensitivity).

We know that 50 patients had an infarction, and 20 did not. So in the above example with a cut-off of 12 µg/1, and two infarction patients missed, sensitivity will equal 48/50, or 0.96 (96%). So 96% of those with an infarction will be correctly identified (two patients with an infarction are missed – false negatives). Specificity will equal 20/20 = 1 or 100%. Twenty patients *don't* have an infarction and *all* will be correctly identified as such. If the cut-off is reduced to 6 µg/1, however, sensitivity increases to 100% (all 50 patients with an infarction are so identified), but specificity is reduced to 50% (10 patients without an infarction are correctly identified, but another 10 are incorrectly diagnosed as having an

Understanding Clinical Papers Second Edition   David Bowers, Allan House, David Owens
© 2006 John Wiley & Sons, Ltd

Comparison of the Effectiveness of Four Clinical Chemical Assays in Classifying Patients with Chest Pain

Andre C. Van Steirteghem,[1] Mark H. Zweig,[2,4] E. Arthur Robertson,[2] Roland M. Bernard,[3] Gustaff Putzeys,[3] and Claude J. Bieva[3]

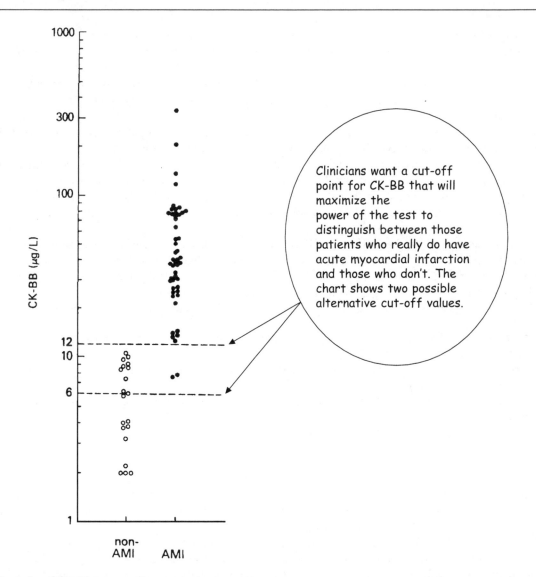

Fig. 2. Serum CK-BB concentrations 16 h after onset of chest pain in patients with (●) and without (○) an AMI

FIGURE 14.1   Serum CK-BB concentrations 16 hours after onset of symptoms in 70 patients presenting with chest pain typical of acute myocardial infarction (AMI)

infarction – false positives). Similar calculations can be performed for the positive predictive value and the negative predictive value.

Clearly, there is an optimal value for the cut-off between sensitivity and specificity which gives the best results for both measures, although this will often be influenced also by the nature of the condition. For example, a diagnostic test for acute myocardial infarction needs as high a sensitivity as possible so that immediate action (aspirin, streptokinase, etc.) can be taken. A high specificity is not so crucial since counter-measures wouldn't harm patients (although it might cause them some alarm). On the other hand, if surgery is the action taken for those identified as having some condition, we would obviously want a very high (preferably 100%) specificity. We don't want to perform invasive procedures on healthy individuals.

We'll come back to this trade-off problem shortly, but for now have a look at Figure 14.2, which is from a validation study for STRATIFY, a risk-of-falling scale for use with elderly hospitalized patients. This scale produces an ordinal risk-of-falling score ranging from 0 to 5 (smaller value means lower risk).

Using cut-off scores of ≥ 2 and ≥ 3, STRATIFY was first applied to a local validation group (similar patients in the same hospital), and then to a sample of similar patients in a different hospital (the remote validation group), and diagnostic performance for each group is shown in the table, along with 95% confidence intervals (we will consider confidence intervals in Chapter 15). You can see the trade-off

Development and evaluation of evidence based risk assessment tool (STRATIFY) to predict which elderly inpatients will fall: case-control and cohort studies

D Oliver, M Britton, P Seed, F C Martin, A H Hopper

Table 3 Usefulness of risk assessment scores of ≥ 2 and ≥ 3 in predicting falls among elderly inpatients in local and remote validation cohorts (phases 2 and 3). Values are percentages (95% confidence intervals)

	Local validation cohort		Remote validation cohort	
	Score ≥ 2	Score ≥ 3	Score ≥ 2	Score ≥ 3
Sensitivity	93.0 (84.3 to 97.7)	69.0 (56.9 to 79.5)	92.4 (84.2 to 97.2)	54.4 (42.8 to 65.7)
Specificity	87.7 (83.6 to 91.0)	96.3 (93.6 to 98.1)	68.3 (63.3 to 73.1)	87.6 (83.8 to 90.8)
Positive predictive value*	62.3 (52.3 to 71.5)	80.3 (68.2 to 89.4)	38.8 (31.8 to 46.2)	48.4 (38.1 to 59.8)
Negative predictive value†	98.3 (96.0 to 99.4)	93.4 (90.2 to 95.8)	97.6 (94.9 to 99.1)	89.9 (86.2 to 92.8)

*Positive predictive value=No of falls with score $\geq n$/No of all scores $\geq n$.
†Negative predictive value=No of falls with score $< n$/No of all scores $< n$.

> Notice in particular the trade-off between sensitivity and specificity values for the different STRATIFY cut-offs ≥ 2 and ≥ 3.

> STRATIFY does not work as well with the remote validation group (possibly due to differences in the two populations).

FIGURE 14.2 Diagnostic test efficacy estimates, using two alternative cut-offs (with 95% confidence intervals) for STRATIFY, a risk assessment tool for detecting potential fallers in an elderly hospital population

between sensitivity and specificity in action – look at the differences in these diagnostics between the ≥ 2 and ≥ 3 cut-offs, sensitivity *decreases* (from 92.4% to 54.4%), while specificity *increases* (from 68.3% to 87.6%). We can also see that, as a diagnostic test, STRATIFY performed less well with the remote group on all measures, but particularly positive predictive value. One possible reason for this is that, although sensitivity and specificity are not affected by the prevalence of the condition in the population, the *predictive* diagnostics PPV and NPV are. If prevalence in the remote validation group was different, we would expect this to alter the PPV and NPV values, as here.

What does all this mean? When you read papers containing diagnostic test studies, you should find information on all four diagnostic measures, along with their confidence intervals, clearly quoted (as an example, see Figure 19.5). If the measure being used for the tests is ordinal or metric, there should be some evidence that various cut-off points have been explored. You also need some information on the prevalence of the condition in the population or populations to which the diagnostic test is applied, particularly if the test is to be used in wider (potentially different) populations.

We now want to return to the sensitivity versus specificity trade-off question. One popular method for finding the optimum cut-off point is to draw a *receiver operating characteristic curve* or ROC curve. This is a plot, for each cut-off point, of sensitivity, the true positive rate, on the vertical axis, against (1 – specificity), the false positive rate, on the horizontal axis. The optimal cut-off is that point on the curve which lies closest to the top left corner. This is also the point which maximises the *area under the curve* (or AUC). In practice, the AUC is calculated (along with its 95% confidence interval) for each cut-off point and the largest value indicates the optimum cut-off.

To see how this works in practice, consider Figure 14.3 which is a receiver operating characteristic curve from a study proposing a new scale (the Psychiatric Symptom Frequency, or PSF, scale) to measure symptoms of anxiety and depression in the UK population. This ROC analysis is for a subgroup of subjects who scored positively on the criterion 'uses prescribed medication'. The 45° diagonal represents a diagnostic test that does not discriminate between those with the condition and those without. The area under the curve for this diagonal line is 0.5. The table below the curve gives the area under the curve value for this ROC curve and two others for different criteria.

If authors have used a receiver operating characteristic curve in their paper, you should see the curve, but certainly be provided with information on the area under it, together with its confidence interval.

As a final point, note that if a test uses a nominal (yes/no) measure – for example, blood in stool (Y/N) – pain when urinating (Y/N), etc., then there can clearly be no trade-off between sensitivity and specificity.

Development of a scale to measure symptoms of anxiety and depression in the general UK population: the psychiatric symptom frequency scale

Malin Lindelow, Rebecca Hardy, Bryan Rodgers

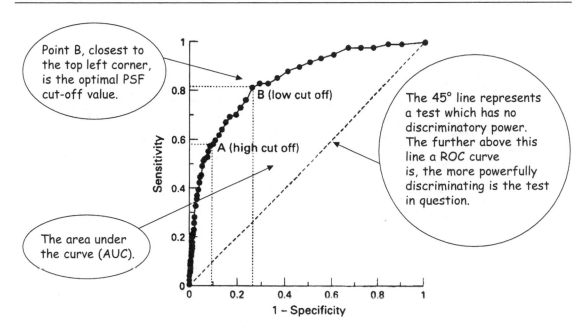

Figure 2   Receiver operating characteristic (ROC) curve for the PSF score where the diagnostic criterion is use of prescribed medication.

Table 1   Results from receiver operating characteristic (ROC) analysis

Criterion variable	Area under curve (SE)	Cut off maximising specificity and sensitivity
Contact with a doctor	0.84 (0.016)	13/14
Use of prescribed medication	0.86 (0.014)	13/14
Suicidal ideation	0.92 (0.012)	19/20

FIGURE 14.3 The receiver operating characteristic curve for each point on the Psychiatric Symptom Frequency scale for subjects who are positive on the criterion 'Taking medication'. The table below the curve shows the area under three ROC/curve, corresponding to subjects who were positive for each of the three criteria shown, along with the standard error (SE). The corresponding confidence intervals are approximately ±2 × SE in each case. The standard error (SE) is a measure of the precision of whichever value is being quoted (here it's the area under the curve AUC). The smaller the SE, the more accurate the value

15

Measurement Scales

At the end of the previous chapter we used an example that described the construction of a scale to measure the frequency of psychiatric symptoms. Clinical papers may often describe the development of a new *measurement scale*, or use data produced by a measurement scale. In this chapter, we are going to say something about these scales, what they are, why they are used, and what qualities we want in a scale.

WHY DO WE NEED MEASUREMENT SCALES?

In Chapter 11, we outlined the difference between categorical data and metric data. Metric variables (such as weight, waiting time, number of deaths, etc.) can be *properly measured*. However, this is not true for categorical variables such as levels of pain or anxiety, degree of well-being, smoking status, ethnic origin, sex, etc.; these have to be *assessed* in some way. For variables such as smoking status or sex, this can be done either by direct observation or questioning. For other variables, like level of depression, degree of general health, predilection for pressure sores, and so on, a different, usually more complex, approach is needed. This usually amounts to using an appropriate measurement scale.

We can illustrate these ideas with the study of low back pain (Figure 12.4). Values for the sociodemographic variables (age, sex, etc.), and the back pain history variables (one or more previous acute episodes, previous chronic episodes) will have been elicited by simple questioning of the patient. However, the *initial disability scores*, and the percentage of subjects suffering *depression and/or generalized anxiety*, will each have been derived from the administration of a measurement scale.

WHAT ARE MEASUREMENT SCALES?

A measurement scale (also referred to as an *instrument*) will usually consist of a questionnaire, or a physical or visual examination, or a mix of these approaches. Some measurement scales are short and reasonably straightforward. For example, the Glasgow Coma Scale has just three questions or *items*: degree of eye opening, of verbal response, and of motor response. Note that in measurement scales the word 'item' is used rather than the word 'question', since the scale may not consist entirely of questions; some observational or measurement elements may be included.

Some scales are longer and more complex and may consist of a number of *dimensions*, each one of which may have one or more items. You can think of each dimension of a scale as a distinct aspect of the condition being measured. For example, a scale to measure general well-being might have three dimensions: physical well-being, mental well-being, and social well-being, each of which might have several questions.

WHEN AUTHORS USE DATA FROM MEASUREMENT SCALES

When authors make use of data derived from a measurement scale they should at least mention the use of the scale in the methods section, and give full source details in the references at the end of the paper.

Understanding Clinical Papers Second Edition   David Bowers, Allan House, David Owens

The authors of the back pain study (Figure 12.4) satisfy this minimum requirement. In their methods section they write, 'Current psychiatric symptoms were investigated by using a structured psychiatric interview based on the DSM-III-R classification flow sheets' and 'Patients filled in a validated French translation of the Roland and Morris disability questionnaire.'

Full source references to both of these instruments are provided in the reference section. On occasion, you might get more detail, for example, a brief description of the structure of the scale being used.

DEVELOPMENT OF A NEW MEASUREMENT SCALE

As well as clinical papers which refer to the use of data from existing scales, you may also encounter papers devoted entirely to the development of a new scale. This can be a complex and lengthy process so what follows is a brief summary.

Researchers will develop a new scale if there is no existing scale that meets their needs. For example, Figure 15.1 is an extract from a paper in which the authors justified the development of a new scale to measure patient satisfaction with nurse-led sexual health clinics because no scale dealing with this area existed. Sometimes an existing scale does exist but is in some way unsuitable, perhaps too long, too expensive, too invasive, or maybe does not quite measure what researchers need to measure. Figure 15.2 is from a paper reporting the development of a new palliative care outcome scale because existing scales did not quite do the job.

Comparing doctor- and nurse-led care in sexual health clinics: patient satisfaction questionnaire

Miles K, Penny N, Power R and Mercy D

… the National Strategy for Sexual Health and HIV proposes that nurses have an expanding role as specialists and consultants for the management of sexually transmitted infections (STIs) …. . However, there is no evidence demonstrating the acceptance of nurses as first-line providers in the speciality of sexual health, or genitourinary medicine (GUM). This paper therefore focuses on an empirical study that aims to develop a *valid and reliable* measure of patient satisfaction that would be used to compare care provided for female patients at nurse-led or doctor-led clinics at a GUM clinic. (our italics)

These authors developed a new scale because there was no existing scale covering this area.

FIGURE 15.1   Development of new scale because there was no suitable existing scale

Development and validation of a core outcome measure for palliative care: the palliative care outcome scale

Hearn J, and Higinson IJ

Quality of life and outcome measures for patients with advanced illness need to be able to assess the key goals of palliative care. Various outcome measures and systems for evaluating palliative care have been developed in recent years. [author then lists a number of such scales].... none of these systematically covers all those domains considered important to palliative care. .... The aim of this study was to develop a core outcome measure for patients with advanced cancer and their families which would cover more than either physical symptoms or quality of life, but remain brief and simple to administer.

These authors developed a new scale because existing scales did not quite do the job.

FIGURE 15.2   Development of new scale because the existing scale didn't quite do the job

SCALE CONSTRUCTION

The construction of a new measurement scale will consist of a number of stages:

- Careful consideration of the condition in question. What is it? How does it arise? How is it manifest? Talking to patients and those familiar and experienced with the condition will be part of this process.
- Research of the literature and examination of any existing scales covering the same or similar conditions.
- The first two stages lead to a tentative initial selection of items which cover the domain of the condition (some of these items may be borrowed from existing scales).
- Once a set of items has been identified, these will need to be put into question form. The authors might refer to questions of some specific format. For example, the authors of a paper describing the development of a new scale to measure the attitudes and beliefs of patients towards hyperlipidemia and its treatments, report that: 'Response categories used a 5-point *Likert scale* to assess the degree to which patients agreed or disagreed with each attitudinal statement.'
- The questions are then organized into an appropriate order and structure – and hence into a scale.
- A draft of the scale can then be passed back to the experienced colleagues who can check that all important aspects of the condition are covered by the suggested items and make suggestions to plug any existing gaps. The object is parsimony, i.e. just enough items to cover the domain adequately, but no more.
- The new scale will then have to be road-tested to ensure that it possesses a number of properties desirable in any scale.

The Likert scale quoted above is one of a number of possible ways of framing questions. Readers who want to know more can refer to *Research Methods in Health* by Ann Bowling (1997), which contains a chapter on this topic.

When they are choosing scale items, you may see authors reporting their use of the techniques of *factor* (or *principal component*) analysis, or less often, of discriminant analysis. These methods are a little too complex to discuss in any detail here, but briefly, factor (or principal component) analysis is a procedure for identifying a smaller number of underlying variables, known as *constructs*, from a larger set of variables.

For example, a patient may experience sweaty palms, nausea, restlessness, loss of appetite, and loss of interest in things previously enjoyed. You might interpret the first three symptoms as a manifestation of underlying anxiety, and the last two as a manifestation of an underlying depression. So the original five variables can be expressed in terms of two underlying factors, which can be interpreted as two separate dimensions.

Discriminant analysis is seen less often but is a way of classifying a number of items into two separate groups.

DESIRABLE PROPERTIES OF SCALES

When you read a clinical paper describing the development of a new scale, the authors need to demonstrate that their scale has a number of properties, without which the scale will be valueless. For example, Figure 15.3 is extracted from a paper which describes the development of a scale to measure children's emotional responses during medical procedures.

Clearly the validity and reliability of a measurement scale are (along with other qualities) important and we want to provide an outline of these and other desirable scale properties. We will do this assuming the scale is questionnaire-based, which most scales are (other than the most simple). Note that there is some inconsistency in the literature in the use of some of the terms used.

Children's Emotional Manifestation Scale: Development and Testing

Ho Cheung W and Lopez V

Therefore there is a need for preoperative interventions that can minimise children's anxiety and enhance their ability to cope with surgery. First, however, to evaluate the effectiveness of preoperative interventions, the availability of a *valid and reliable* instrument that accurately documents the manifestation of children's emotions towards stressful medical procedures is crucial. Regrettably, the existing literature lacks an assessment tool with effective properties. (our italics)

It is important that any measurement scale is both valid and reliable.

FIGURE 15.3   The scale properties of validity and reliability in a scale to measure children's emotions

Scale Validity

Put simply, *validity* is the ability of a scale to measure what it is supposed to measure, no more or no less. You will see references to a number of different 'types' of validity, the most important of which we will now describe.

Face Validity

If a scale appears on the surface to be measuring what it is supposed to be measuring, and does so with simple, relevant, and unambiguous questions, then it is said to have the property of *face validity*. This property is thought to increase the level of compliance of those completing the questionnaire.

Clinical papers may report a number of ways in which face validity might be checked, although none of these should present any difficulty in understanding. Many researchers use *reading* simplicity. For example, to quote again from the hyperlipidemia medication adherence paper, the scale questions were evaluated and,

> This activity resulted in the re-wording, and sometimes the elimination, of poorly or awkwardly worded items, or items that were judged to be poor representatives of their constructs. The items as a whole were also reviewed in terms of readability. The Flesch–Kinkaid reading grade level rated the final survey at a 6th grade level. (That is, the reading ability of 12-year-olds.)

And from the paper on the development of a patient satisfaction questionnaire for patients attending a sexual health clinic: 'The second draft of the questionnaire was viewed for face validity with nine patients of various ethnic origins and ages. Difficult questions were reworded and ambiguous questions excluded.'

Content Validity

Roughly speaking, a scale has *content validity* if there are enough items in the scale to address adequately the domain of the construct (the aspect of the condition) in question. In other words, all the items in the scale are relevant to the construct and all aspects of the construct are covered by the items in the scale. A scale with content validity measures what it is supposed to measure (and it doesn't measure what it is not supposed to).

For example, the Pressure Sore Prediction Score scale (PSPS) has six dimensions, each with only one item, and this is considered by the scale's designers to be sufficient to completely describe the domain of 'getting a pressure sore'. These dimensions and their items are as follows:

1. Does the patient sit up in bed?
2. Is the patient unconscious?
3. Is the patient in poor general condition?
4. Is the patient incontinent?
5. Can the patient lift up from the bed?
6. Does the patient get up and walk around?

The author believes that this scale has content validity (although does not demonstrate that it does!). So in inference terms, the higher a patient's score on this scale, the more confident we can be that that patient will develop a pressure sore. Notice that the designer of this scale did not consider it necessary to have, say, an age or skin condition item.

In comparison, the Waterlow Pressure Sore Risk Assessment Scale has both skin condition and age (as well as sex), in a six-dimension, 32-item scale. Clearly a scale which is missing some important aspect of the condition being assessed is likely to produce less satisfactory results, i.e. less reliable inferences, when its scores are used for prediction.

Ensuring that a scale has content validity needs careful item selection and is part of the scale development process. Some authors might demonstrate that their scale has this property. How? One accepted method is to ask a number of experienced specialists to review the scale and rate the relevancy of each item. For example, in their paper describing the development of their children's emotional scale (referred to above), content validity is demonstrated as follows:

> Content validity was established by six nurse experts rating of each item on a four-point scale (from 1 = not relevant to 4 = very relevant). The Content Validity Index (CVI), the % of the total number of items rated by the experts as either 3 or 4, was 96%. A CVI score of 80% or higher is generally considered to have good content validity.

Criterion or Concurrent Validity

Suppose there exists a well-established 'gold standard' or *criterion* scale used for measuring anxiety, but it is long, and thus time-consuming and expensive to administer. If a new, shorter scale is developed whose results agree or correlate well with the criterion scale when they are both administered to the same group of subjects *at the same time* (which is the *concurrent* bit), then the new scale is said to have the property of *criterion or concurrent* validity. In which case, it may be substituted for the existing scale (provided it is otherwise satisfactory). We will deal with the idea of *correlation* as a measure of the association between two variables more fully in Chapter 22.

Thus authors might demonstrate that their new scale has criterion validity by showing that their new scale agrees strongly with the gold standard scale – if an alternative gold standard scale is available. Unfortunately this is not usually the case. For example, on the development of a patient satisfaction questionnaire for patients at a sexual health clinic, the authors comment:

> Concurrent validity could involve the questionnaire being administered alongside an existing measure to determine whether there was a strong correlation between the two. Since no measure of satisfaction relevant to sexual health was identified, a comparative measure against another scale was not possible.

Authors may sometimes mention a variant of criterion validity known as *predictive validity*. This scale property relates to situations where the criterion, against which we want to judge our new scale, may not be available until some time has passed. For example, we may have a scale which indicates something which can only be confirmed (or not) with a biopsy. If the usual situation prevails – no suitable criterion scale exists – then criterion validity obviously cannot be established. In these circumstances, researchers may turn to construct validity.

Construct Validity

We cannot directly measure things such as anxiety, well-being, the likelihood of pressure sores, and so on, in the same way we can measure temperature or systolic blood pressure. We can of course assess the various *surface* manifestations of anxiety – sweaty palms, restlessness, nausea, and so on – without too much difficulty. Underlying conditions, such as anxiety or well-being, are known *constructs*, and many scales are designed to measure them. For a scale to have *construct validity*, it must provide a true assessment of the existence and level of the construct in question. If authors of a clinical paper are describing the development of a new scale, they should demonstrate that their scale has construct validity. There are a number of ways in which they can do this which may be referred to in scale development papers.

One possibility is for them to make hypotheses about the responses of subjects to their new scale and demonstrate that these hypotheses are satisfied. These hypotheses might include a comparison of their scale with an existing scale which purports to measure the same construct, for example, by examining correlations between scores, which should be reasonably high. Conversely, they may compare their scale with another scale which should *not* be related. These would be expected to produce non-significant or even negative correlations, for example, applying an anxiety scale to calm and relaxed individuals.

Another possibility is for authors to apply the new scale to two groups, one group believed to have the condition or construct, the other group not (this approach is known as the *method of extreme groups*). The first group should produce low scores on the new scale, the second group high scores. A further possibility might be to give a therapeutic intervention to the same two dissimilar groups, who might be expected to react differently if the scale is a good measure of the underlying construct.

Figure 15.4 is from a study into the use of the SF36 scale to measure the general health of post-stroke patients (the authors claiming that this application of SF36 was unexplored). This is an example of the scale comparison method of establishing construct validity. The authors compared their proposed scale with a number of other scales, first making hypotheses about the expected correlations. Figure 15.5 shows the authors' comment taken from their results section. They do not comment further as to whether or not they feel these results establish construct validity.

As a final comment, it is important to note that a scale developed for some particular population, even with large and representative samples, and whose validity has been satisfactorily demonstrated (we might describe it as being *internally* valid), may not be *externally* valid, i.e. it may not be valid when applied to some different population.

RELIABILITY

Even before the validity of a new scale is ensured, its *reliability* must first be established. Simply put, reliability means that the scale has the property of *repeatability or reproducibility*. You can administer it any number of times and it will always give consistent results. In other words, when a reliable scale is applied to a group of individuals by a single observer at two different times, or by two observers at the same time, it will produce *similar* scores. The crucial word here is 'similar'. How close do the scores have to be before they can be judged to be similar and the scale thus said to be reliable?

The authors of any scale development paper should demonstrate that their scale is reliable. You are unlikely to see anything like a 'reliability coefficient' quoted. Instead, authors may report a number of reliability-associated measures, the more important ones which we describe briefly below. As you will see, the similarity between scores can be judged in a number of ways.

Internal consistency – Cronbach's α

Internal consistency is one measure thought to reflect the reliability of a scale. You might expect that a scale addressing some underlying construct will have a number of similar items. For example, the Geriatric Depression Scale (GDS) has questions like, 'Have you dropped many of your activities and interests?' 'Do you feel that your life is empty?', 'Do you often feel helpless?', and so on. These questions are clearly tapping into the same construct. It seems reasonable to expect that if the test is

Psychometric properties of the SF36 in the early post-stroke phase

Hagen S, Bugge C and Alexander H

Construct validity was assessed by examining the relationship between the eight SF36 subscores and the scores on other standard outcome measures: the Barthel Activities of Daily Living (ADL) Index, the Canadian Neurological Scale (CNS), and the Mini-Mental State Examination (MMSE). …. On the basis of the content of the questions it was hypothesised that there would be positive bivariate correlations between all SF36 subscores and the Barthel Index, MMSE and CNS. … The latter three instruments, used here for validation purposes, all measure some aspect of physical or cognitive ability which should be associated, directly or indirectly, with elements of health status measured within the SF36. More specifically, we would expect only low to moderate correlations between SF36 scores and the MMSE as the SF36 items do not directly address cognitive problems. In general, higher correlation coefficients would be expected in relation to the Barthel Index and the CNS which address physical aspects of health and related disability. The highest correlations might be expected between Physical Functioning, Role Limitation - Physical, General Health, and Social Functioning scores and both the Barthel and CNS. Moderate correlations might be expected between Bodily Pain, Vitality, and Role Limitation – Emotional scores and the Barthel Index and CNS. It was expected that Mental Health scores would be weakly correlated with the Barthel Index, CNS and MMSE scores. Spearman's rank correlations were used to test for associations.

The authors of this paper tested for the construct validity of SF36 in post-stroke patients by comparing SF36 scores with the Barthel ADL Index, the MMSE and the Canadian Neurological Scale. They hypothesised various levels of correlation between SF36 and these three other scales.

FIGURE 15.4 Demonstrating construct validity, from a paper on the use of SF36 with post-stroke patients (Note: Physical Functioning, Role Limitation – Physical, General Health, Social Functioning, Bodily Pain, Vitality, Role Limitation – Emotional, and Mental Health, are all dimensions of SF36.)

reliable, then the scores by a group of patients on one of these items will be correlated with their scores on other, similar, items.

Such correlations are said to measure *internal consistency*, and one common method of measuring this correlation is with *Cronbach's alpha* (α). To be acceptable, α should have a value above 0.7. One problem with α is that it is dependent on the number of items in the scale. Increase the number of items and α will increase (although the actual inter-item correlations may not have changed!). A second problem is that α takes no account of variation from observer to observer, or from one time period to another, and is thus likely to exaggerate reliability.

As an example from the literature, the authors of a paper describing the development of a scale to measure the attitudes of nurses working with acute mental health patients, the Attitudes Towards Acute Mental Health Scale (ATAMHS), reported the reliability of their scale as follows: 'The sample obtained for this study was greater than the 100 participants regarded as the minimum to ensure reliability of the

Psychometric properties of the SF 36 in the early post-stroke phase

Hagen S, Bugge C and Alexander H

The strongest correlations were found between SF36 scores and the Barthel Index and CNS, as hypothesised. The highest of these were with Physical Functioning and Social Functioning as expected; however, correlations with Role Limitations – Physical was markedly lower … . Correlations with Mental Health scores were stronger than expected for both the Barthel Index and CNS. Correlations between SF36 and MMSE scores were moderate for Physical Functioning and Mental Health and weaker for the remaining subscales, as expected.

The results of the author's comparisons of their scale and three other scales as a measure of construct validity.

FIGURE 15.5   Authors' comment on the correlations between scale scores from the paper shown in Figure 15.4 on the use of the SF36 scale with post-stroke patients

statistical procedures.… The ATAMHS had a coefficient alpha of 0.72, which indicated reasonable reliability.' Similarly, the authors of the post-stroke SF36 study, referred to earlier, reported the reliability of the SF36 scale thus:

> The reliability of the SF36 was assessed in terms of it's internal consistency. … all values of Cronbach's α exceeded the generally accepted criterion of 0.7. This would tend to indicate a high level of correlation among items within the same subscale, and correspondingly good reliability.

Internal consistency can also be thought of as a measure of the *homogeneity* of a scale. By this, we mean that all the items in a scale should be addressing different aspects of the same underlying construct, and not different constructs. For example, if we are measuring some particular phobia, then all the scale items should relate in some way to different aspects of this phobia, not to other phobias or other general anxieties or fears. The implication of homogeneity is that all the items should correlate to some extent with each other, and should also correlate with the total scale score. As you have just seen, this is the basis of measures of internal consistency. This notion leads to the idea of *split-half reliability*. This involves splitting the scale items randomly into two equal halves and then correlating the two halves. If the scale is internally consistent, then the two halves should be strongly correlated, and hence reliable.

Stability

The *stability* of a measurement scale is a further measure of its reliability. This is the capacity of a scale to give similar scores in the following situations:

- when administered to a particular group of individuals at different time periods – *test–retest* reliability;
- when administered by two different observers – *inter-observer* reliability;
- when administered by the same observer at two different time periods – *intra-observer* reliability.

Reproducibility of the University of Toronto Self-administered Questionnaire Used to Assess Environmental Sensitivity

McKeown-Eyssen GE, Sokoloff ER, Jazmaji V, Marshall LM and Baines CJ

Reproducibility of the questionnaire was assessed by comparing responses from people who completed it on two different occasions. …. Within 5-7 months of returning the first questionnaire 200 respondents were randomly selected to receive the questionnaire a second time …. Kappa statistics were statistically significant for all systems (13 body systems were monitored), and were above 0.4 for 11 of 13 systems, indicating good levels of agreement. (and thus of test–retest reliability)

The first three lines of the authors' results are shown below:

Body system	% observed agreement	kappa	95% CI
Eye	88.8	0.57	0.37, 0.76
Ear	79.1	0.53	0.38, 0.68
Nose	89.6	0.36	0.13, 0.62

These authors used kappa to measure the test–retest stability (and thus the reliability) of their environment sensitivity scale.

FIGURE 15.6   Using kappa to examine the test – retest (reliability) property of scale

As far as test–retest reliability is concerned, the clinical paper should tell you how long the interval is between the first administration of the test and the second – two to 14 days is usual, although longer periods might be acceptable depending on the condition being measured.

All three of these forms of stability-reliability are probably best measured by the *intraclass correlation coefficient* (ICC). In practice, perhaps because the ICC is not always readily computable, authors may present a value either for a correlation coefficient, or for Cohen's chance-adjusted coefficient of agreement, kappa (κ), which we will discuss in more detail in Chapter 23. Briefly, kappa measures the agreement between two sets of scores discounting any element of agreement expected to have arisen by chance.

An example of test–retest stability (and hence scale reliability) which uses kappa is shown in Figure 15.6. This is from a study into the reproducibility of a scale to assess environmental sensitivity in individuals exposed to a range of substances in the environment.

Figure 15.7 is an example of test–retest stability which uses correlation. This is from the previously quoted study on a scale to measure patient satisfaction with nurse-led sexual health clinics (see Figure 15.1).

Comparing doctors and nurse-led care in sexual health clinics: patient satisfaction questionaire

Miles K, Perry N, Power R and Mercy D

Phase 6 – test-retest stability

The final questionnaire consisted of 34 statements. It was re-administered (n=28) in the clinic, and 13 women agreed to receive a second postal questionnaire. …. with a mean of 13.75 days between first and second questionnaires . The second questionnaire was used to confirm stability, using a test-retest analysis. …. A Pearson correlation between the original and re-test scores was 0.95 (p<0.001), demonstrating questionnaire stability.

These authors used Pearson correlation to measure the test-retest stability (and thus the reliability) of their patient satisfaction scale.

FIGURE 15.7   Using correlation to examine the test – retest (reliability) property of a patient satisfaction scale for use in sexual health clinics

A value of 0.95 for Pearson's correlation coefficient indicates a very strong association between the original scores and the retest scores. Note however that the sample size is very small which makes for unreliable results, and in addition, as you will see in Chapter 22, for ordinal data such as this, Spearman's correlation coefficient is more appropriate.

SENSITIVITY TO CHANGE – SCALE RESPONSIVENESS

If we are interested in the effect of some therapeutic intervention on a group of individuals suffering from some condition, then we want the scale which measures that condition to be sensitive to any change due to the intervention. In other words we want the scale to be able to capture the *treatment effect*. We call this the *sensitivity-to-change* or *responsiveness* property of the scale. In any paper describing the development of such a scale the authors should demonstrate that it has this property.

One way that they might do this is to measure changes over some time period using both their new scale and some other comparable scales. Ideally these comparisons will be not only with scales which might be expected to reflect *similar* change, but also with scales which should not. What actual method is used for the comparison will depend on the particular circumstances – on the nature of the data for example – but correlation is one possibility.

Notice that there is a tension between the sensitivity-to-change property of a scale and the idea of test – retest reliability. Clearly, the latter is not appropriate for conditions where there is likely to be change over the short term, particularly where any therapeutic intervention is envisaged, and certainly not during the test – retest interval.

As an example of scale sensitivity to change we can return again to the study using SF36 with post-stroke patients (see Figure 15.4). One of the stated aims of this study was, 'To examine the reliability, validity and *sensitivity to change* of the SF36 in patients in the early post-stroke period' (our italics). SF36 scores were measured at 1, 3 and 6 months post-stroke. Figure 15.8 is an extract from that paper in

Psychometric properties of the SF36 in the early post-stroke phase

Hagen S, Bugge C and Alexander H

Significant improvements were seen between 1 and 3 months in all SF36 subscores except Bodily Pain, General Health, and Mental Health. Similarly there were significant improvements in Barthel Index, CNS and MMSE scores. There were no significant changes in SF36 scores between 3 and 6 months while, of the three comparison measures, the CNS and MMSE both showed significant improvement. .... Between 3 and 6 months, none of the SF36 subscales appeared to be responsive to change.

The authors measured sensitivity to change of SF36 in post-stroke patients by comparing change over time in SF36 with change in three other scales.

FIGURE 15.8   Sensitivity to change of SF36 in post-stroke patients

which the authors used Wilcoxon's matched-pairs test to compare median change scores between a number of SF36 sub-scales, and the Barthel Activities of Daily Living (ADL) Index, the Canadian Neurological Scale (CNS), and the Mini-Mental State Examination (MMSE). The authors concluded that, 'Sensitivity to change was poorer in the later stages of the study.'

THE USE OF ROC CURVES WITH SCALE SCORES

Finally, authors may mention the use of the ROC curve in conjunction with their newly developed scale as a way of determining optimum cut-off points for the scores obtained from it. The use of ROC curves and the sensitivity/specificity of cut-off scores were described in Chapter 14.

Establishing More of the Facts:
Some Common Ways of Describing Results

16

Fractions, Proportions and Rates

Researchers often present their findings as raw numbers, but it may be that more sense is conveyed when the raw number becomes some kind of fraction. Probably the most widely used fractions in health research are *proportions*. Proportions are fractions in which the numerator (the bit on the top) is a subset of the denominator (remember that in the fraction ¾, 3 is called the numerator and 4 is called the denominator). For example, ¾ could mean 3 out of 4; if so, then it is a proportion. Proportions can be useful because they allow various judgements and comparisons that are not possible with raw numbers.

If, for example, the annual number of adults who attend an accident and emergency department after harming themselves (usually by self-poisoning with medicines of some kind) rises over a 5-year period from 850 to 1350, the rise is by more than 50%. However, the number of adults in the catchment population may also have risen over the same period. Consequently, when the yearly proportions of adults attending are calculated, the apparent increase in self-harm might be much smaller, say, from 280 to 350 per 100 000. In health research a common explanation for an increase in denominator is an alteration in the catchment population served by the hospital (perhaps, in this example, when a nearby accident and emergency department closed down).

A more complex fraction commonly used in research is a *rate*. A rate has a numerator, a denominator and a stated time period: for example, 10 suicides per 100 000 persons (of all ages) per year is the approximate suicide rate in England and Wales at the time of writing. One widely used rate in clinical epidemiology is the *inception rate* (also known as *incidence*) of a disease, referring to the rate of new cases arising. If the inception rate for schizophrenia is around 2 per 10 000 per year, then a city of half a million might expect 100 new cases each year. Motor neurone disease has a much lower estimated incidence: around 2 per 100 000 per year.

The *prevalence* of a disease usually refers to the number of existing cases at the time of counting; it therefore includes those who have long since developed the disease as well as more recent cases. For long-lasting conditions prevalence is much higher than incidence. For example, motor neurone disease has a prevalence of around 7 per 100 000. Chronic but not life-threatening diseases such as rheumatoid arthritis have even larger differences between incidence and prevalence. Because it is not defined by duration, prevalence is not really a rate but a proportion, although it is common to see it mistakenly referred to as 'prevalence rate'.

Sometimes you will see a prevalence described as a *period prevalence* or a *point prevalence*. If we collected all of the cases present in a particular population at one point in time (sometimes called a *census date*), that would give us a point prevalence. If we collected all the cases present during a particular period of time, say, a month or a year, that would give us a period prevalence. Period prevalence will include all new cases arising in that period as well as all cases that existed at the start of the period and extend into it. For relatively chronic and stable conditions (like multiple sclerosis, for example), point prevalence is a good measure, while for more transient disorders (like, say, back pain bad enough to lead to time off work), a period prevalence may give a better measure of burden to the community.

Figure 16.1 is part of the abstract of a study about trends in self-harm. The study is full of raw numbers that have been turned into various proportions and rates. In practice, we often want to examine

Understanding Clinical Papers Second Edition   David Bowers, Allan House, David Owens
© 2006 John Wiley & Sons, Ltd

Trends in deliberate self-harm in Oxford, 1985–1995

Implications for clinical services and the prevention of suicide

KEITH HAWTON, JOAN FAGG, SUE SIMKIN, ELIZABETH BALE
and ALISON BOND

Background Deliberate self-harm (DSH) has been a major health problem in the UK for nearly three decades. Any changes in rates of DSH or the demographic characteristics of the patient population are likely to have important implications for clinical services and suicide prevention.

Method Data collected by the Oxford Monitoring System for Attempted Suicide were used to review trends in DSH between 1985–1995.

Results There was a substantial increase in DSH rates during the 11-year study period, with a 62.1% increase in males and a 42.2% increase in females. The largest rise was in 15–24-year-old males (+194.1%). Changes in DSH rates correlated with changes in national suicide rates in both males and females in this age group. Rates of repetition of DSH increased in both genders during the study period. Paracetamol self-poisoning has continued to increase, half of all overdoses in 1995 involving paracetamol, and antidepressant overdoses have become more common.

Rates are compared year by year over 11 years. Raw numbers of persons carrying out self-harm might be misleading because of population change.

This age-and-sex-specific rate reveals a key finding: it was the young men who largely accounted for the rise in self-harm rate. The authors add (not shown here) that rates in other male age groups did not rise sharply.

We need this simple *proportion* rather than raw numbers of paracetamol overdoses to judge whether something is going on.

FIGURE 16.1   Summary of a descriptive study setting out relevant rates and proportions

rates according to a variety of denominators. In the text (but not shown here in the abstract) these authors describe a 51% increase in the self-harm rate during the study period (called an increase in 'crude rate'); in figure 16.1 they set out rates for males and females ('sex-specific rates') and for 15–24-year-old males (an 'age-and-sex-specific rate').

17

Risk and Odds

If you toss a coin you know the chance of it coming down heads. People use various ways to express this chance (Figure 17.1). Notice that, strangely, the ways of describing the chance split into those that yield a numerical result of a half and those with a numerical result of one. This is because in practice we use two quite different fractions to express chance: *risk* and *odds*. For most of us, risk accords with the way we think in our everyday lives and is much the easier to understand. Researchers, however, calculate and tell readers about chance in terms of risks *and* odds, so this chapter sets out the principles of both these expressions of chance.

One in two	Evens
Fifty per cent (50%)	One-to-one
0.5	Fifty-fifty
A half	Equal chance
Expressed numerically as 0.5	Expressed numerically as 1

FIGURE 17.1 Terminology in common use when describing the chance of tossing a head

Suppose you tossed a coin twice and it came down once as a head and once as a tail. This is represented in Figure 17.2. Looking at Figure 17.2, you might reasonably say that the *risk* (or probability) of tossing a head is: Heads (1) divided by the total of Heads and Tails (2), which comes out at $1/2 = 0.5$. The risk can be described as a fraction in which the numerator corresponds to the number of times an event occurs while the denominator corresponds to the total number of possible events. The *odds* of tossing a head, however, is rather different: you divide Heads (1) by Tails (1) – which comes out at $1/1 = 1$. The odds, therefore, can be described as a fraction in which the numerator corresponds to the number of times an event occurs while the denominator corresponds to the number of times an event does not occur. If you look back at Figure 17.1 you should now be able to make sense of the two sets of terms: the terms in the left-hand column refer to risk, those on the right to odds.

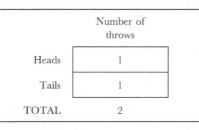

	Number of throws
Heads	1
Tails	1
TOTAL	2

FIGURE 17.2 A plausible result from two tosses of a coin

RISK

In clinical research, risk has the same meaning as *probability*; the terminology has been heavily influenced by public health academics who have concentrated on the concept of *risk factors* causing disease. One

Understanding Clinical Papers Second Edition   David Bowers, Allan House, David Owens
© 2006 John Wiley & Sons, Ltd

consequence of risk and probability being synonyms is that it is accepted practice to refer to the risk of bad or good events occurring. For example, researchers may calculate and tell you the risk of getting better from a disease; in epidemiological terms risk doesn't necessarily carry the connotation of danger.

ODDS

Odds is (or *odds are*; it's accepted practice to speak of odds as plural or singular) another bona fide method of expressing chance. Although most people find risk easier to think about, odds has several properties that are invaluable to epidemiologists and statisticians. It is not important here to go into why odds is such a useful measure, but one of the main reasons is explained in Chapter 18, where we describe the calculation and uses of *risk ratios* and *odds ratios*.

Extracts from the two papers in Figures 17.3 and 17.4 illustrate the use of the fractions *risk* and *odds*. In each case the authors want us to infer a connection between some variable and the subsequent development of a condition.

Change in social status and risk of low birth weight in Denmark: population based cohort study

Olga Basso, Jørn Olsen, Anne Mette T Johansen, Kaare Christensen

---

Abstract

Objective: To estimate the risk of having a low birth-weight infant associated with changes in social, environmental, and genetic factors.
Design: Population based, historical cohort study using the Danish medical birth registry and Statistic Denmark's fertility database.
Subjects: All women who had a low birthweight infant (<2500 g) (index birth) and a subsequent liveborn infant (outcome birth) in Denmark between 1980 and 1992 (exposed cohort, n = 11 069) and a random sample of the population who gave birth to an infant weighing ≥2500 g and to a subsequent liveborn infant (unexposed cohort, n = 10 211).
Main outcome measures: Risk of having a low birthweight infant in the outcome birth as a function of changes in male partner, area of residence, type of job, and social status between the two births.
Results: Women in the exposed cohort showed a high risk (18.5%) of having a subsequent low birthweight infant while women in the unexposed cohort had a risk of 2.8%. After adjustment for initial social status, a decline in social status increased the absolute risk of having a low birthweight infant by about 5% in both cohorts, though this was significantly only in the unexposed cohort. Change of male partner did not modify the risk of low birth weight in either cohort.
Conclusion: Having had a low birthweight infant and a decline in social status are strong risk factors for having a low birthweight infant subsequently.

> Here the researchers are interested in the risk of a subsequent low birthweight infant if a previous childbirth was of low weight.

> They determine this risk and compare it with the equivalent risk in a general population sample.

FIGURE 17.3   Determining risk in a cohort study

Helicobacter pylori infection and mortality from ischaemic heart disease: negative result from a large, prospective study

N J Wald, M R Law, J K Morris, A M Bagnall

Abstract

Objective—To determine whether there is an independent association between *Helicobacter pylori* infection of the stomach and ischaemic heart disease.
Design—Prospective study with measurement of IgG antibody titres specific to *H pylori* on stored serum samples from 648 men who died from ischaemic heart disease and 1296 age matched controls who did not (nested case-control design).
Subjects—21 520 professional men aged 35–64 who attended the British United Provident Association (BUPA) medical centre in London between 1975 and 1982 for routine medical examination.
Main outcome measure—Death from ischaemic heart disease.
Results—The odds of death from ischaemic heart disease in men with *H pylori* infection relative to that in men without infection was 1.06 (95% confidence interval 0.86 to 1.31). In a separate group of 206 people attending the centre, plasma fibrinogen was virtually the same in those who were positive for *H pylori* (2.62 g/l) and those who were negative (2.64 g/l).

Men with or without *Helicobacter pylori* infection are compared as to their odds of developing a myocardial infarction. The authors chose to compare the two odds, but could as easily have calculated the two risks (one for each group) and compared those.

The authors divide the two odds to find the value 1.06: the odds of death for men with the disease relative to the odds of death for men without the disease. This is the odds ratio (discussed in Chapter 18).

FIGURE 17.4 Determining odds (expressed as one odds relative to another) in a cohort study

18

Ratios of Risk and Odds

RISK RATIO (RELATIVE RISK)

You were introduced to the calculation of risks in Chapter 17. This chapter deals with the issues of risk ratios and odds ratios. Researchers in Italy examined evidence that suggested that women with breast cysts might be susceptible to breast cancer (Figure 18.1). They investigated the hypothesis that the chemical composition of the fluid that can be aspirated from a cyst (using a needle and syringe) provides a clue to cancer risk. The women in their study, as part of a breast cancer detection programme, were all followed up for between 2 and 12 years. Using a cohort analytic study design (see Chapter 5), the researchers compared the proportions of women who developed breast cancer among those who had Type I cysts (high concentration of potassium, low concentrations of sodium and chloride) and those shown to have Type II cysts (low concentration of potassium, high concentrations of sodium and chloride).

The researchers here have calculated that the risk of cancer among the women with Type I cysts is 12 divided by 417 = 0.029 (or 2.9%). The risk of cancer among the women with Type II cysts is 2 divided by 325 = 0.0062 (or 0.62%). A popular approach to summarizing these kinds of findings, which the authors have used here, is the *risk ratio* (also known as the *relative risk*). It is a comparison of these two risks – arrived at by dividing one by the other: 2.9 divided by 0.62 = 4.7.

If, for simplicity, we round this risk ratio up to 5, then we might say that the women with Type I cysts have about a five times greater risk of breast cancer than do the women with Type II cysts. Another correct and readily comprehensible way of expressing the finding is to say that breast cancer is five times more likely in the women with Type I cysts (compared with those with Type II cysts).

By the same logic, if the risks were identical in the two study groups being compared, the risk ratio would be 1. Risk ratios below 1 indicate that the characteristic under scrutiny confers less rather than more risk. Here the authors could have divided 0.62 by 2.9 (which comes to about 0.2) and thereby reported something like: 'the incidence of breast cancer in women with Type II cysts was lower than in women with Type I cysts (relative risk 0.2)'. Of course, 0.2 is the same thing as one-fifth; if the first group has one-fifth the risk of the second group, it is tantamount to saying that the second has five times the risk of the first. In other words, it is acceptable to express the risk ratio either way so long as you are careful with the wording.

The two terms 'risk ratio' and 'relative risk' are widely used. We prefer *risk ratio* because it mirrors what happens with odds in the odds ratio (see below). Chapter 20 describes how confidence intervals are applied to the risk ratio.

ODDS RATIO

Back in Chapter 17, dealing with odds and risk, we tried to demonstrate that the chance of something happening could reasonably be expressed as a risk or as an odds. No surprise then that the *odds ratio* is used to compare two odds in a way that mirrors calculation of the risk ratio for the comparison of two risks.

Back in Italy, but further south in Naples, another research team investigated whether children who experienced a febrile convulsion might be anaemic. The factors that determine why some children suffer

Understanding Clinical Papers Second Edition   David Bowers, Allan House, David Owens
© 2006 John Wiley & Sons, Ltd

Cohort study of association of risk of breast cancer with cyst type in women with gross cystic disease of the breast

Paolo Bruzzi, Luigi Dogliotti, Carlo Naldoni, Lauro Bucchi, Massimo Costantini, Alessandro Cicognani, Mirella Torta, Gian Franco Buzzi, Alberto Angeli

Abstract

Objective: To assess correlation between type of breast cyst and risk of breast cancer in women with gross cystic disease of the breast.

Design: Cohort study of women with breast cysts aspirated between 1983 and 1993 who were followed up until December 1994 for occurrence of breast cancer.

Setting: Major cancer prevention centre.

Subjects: 802 women with aspirated breast cysts.

Main outcome measures: Type of breast cyst based on cationic content of cyst fluid: type I (potassium:sodium ratio >1.5), type II (potassium:sodium ratio <1.5), or mixed (both types). Subsequent occurrence and type of breast cancer.

Results: After median follow up of six years (range 2–12 years) 15 cases of invasive breast cancer and two ductal carcinomas in situ were diagnosed in the cohort: 12 invasive cancers (and two carcinomas in situ) among the 417 women with type I cysts, two cancers among the 325 women with type II cysts, and one among the 60 women with mixed cysts. The incidence of breast cancer in women with type I cysts was significantly higher than that in women with type II cysts (relative risk 4.62 (95% confidence interval 1.26 to 29.7). These results were confirmed after adjustment for several risk factors for breast cancer (relative risk 4.24 (1.12 to 27.5)).

Conclusions: The increased risk of breast cancer of women with breast cysts seems to be concentrated among women with type I breast cysts.

Design of cohort studies is described in Chapter 5. They commonly report their findings as risk ratios (relative risks).

12 of 417 women with Type I cysts developed cancer (a risk of 2.9%) . . .

. . . while only 2 of 325 women with Type II cysts developed cancer (a risk of 0.62%).

2.9 divided by 0.62 is 4.6, the *risk ratio* (or *relative risk*).

Chapter 20 describes how confidence intervals are applied to the risk ratio.

Chapters 23–25 deal with adjusting for confounders.

Table 3 Relative risk of invasive breast cancer among 802 women with gross cystic disease by type of breast cyst and number of cysts aspiration at enrolment

	No of subjects	No of cases of cancer	Relative risk (95% CI)	
			Univariate analysis	Multivariate analysis[†]
Type of breast cyst*:				
Type II	325	2	1.00	1.00
Type I	417	12	4.62 (1.26 to 29.7)	4.24 (1.12 to 27.5)
Mixed	60	1	2.57 (0.12 to 26.9)	1.98 (0.07 to 34.4)
No of cysts aspirated:				
Solitary	682	12	1.00	1.00
Multiple	120	3	1.35 (0.31 to 4.24)	1.26 (0.19 to 4.75)

*See text for details of cyst types.
†Adjusted for age, age at menarche, No of births, and family history of breast cancer.

FIGURE 18.1 Summary of a cohort analytic study where the main finding is set out in terms of a risk ratio (relative risk)

Iron deficiency anaemia and febrile convulsions: case–control study in children under 2 years

Alfredo Pisacane, Renato Sansone, Nicola Impagliazzo, Angelo Coppola, Paolo Rolando, Alfonso D'Apuzzo, Ciro Tregrossi

> Case-control studies were described in Chapter 5. They nearly always report their findings as odds ratios.

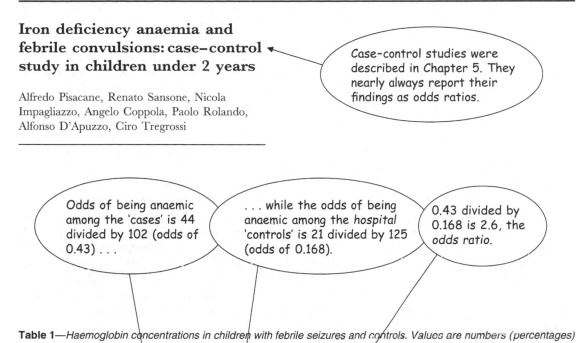

> Odds of being anaemic among the 'cases' is 44 divided by 102 (odds of 0.43) . . .

> . . . while the odds of being anaemic among the *hospital* 'controls' is 21 divided by 125 (odds of 0.168).

> 0.43 divided by 0.168 is 2.6, the *odds ratio.*

Table 1—*Haemoglobin concentrations in children with febrile seizures and controls. Values are numbers (percentages)*

Haemoglobin concentration (g/l)	No (%) of cases (n=146)	Hospital controls		Population controls	
		No (%) (n=146)	Odds ratio (95% confidence interval)	No (%) (n=147)	Odds ratio (95% confidence interval)
≥105	102 (70)	125 (86)	1	130 (88.4)	1
<105	44 (30)	21 (14)	2.6 (1.4 to 4.8)	17 (11.6)	3.3 (1.7 to 6.5)

> Chapter 20 describes how confidence intervals are applied to odds ratios.

FIGURE 18.2   Table from a case–control study where the main findings are set out in terms of odds ratios

(see Chapter 5) the researchers measured the haemoglobin levels of 146 consecutive children admitted to their hospital as a consequence of a febrile seizure (Figure 18.2). They compared haemoglobin levels for the children who had seizures with haemoglobin levels for children in two 'control' groups (who had not had seizures): first, a random sample of 146 children admitted to the same ward but with respiratory or gastrointestinal infections, and second, a random sample of 147 healthy children drawn from the provincial birth register. The table sets out their main findings.

Among the 146 'cases' of children who had seizures, the odds of being anaemic (having a haemoglobin level below 105 grammes per litre) is 44 divided by 102 = 0.43. The odds of being anaemic for those in the *hospital* control group is 21 divided by 125 = 0.168. The odds ratio comparison of these two odds – arrived at by dividing one by the other – is 0.43 divided by 0.168 = 2.6. The odds ratio to compare cases with the *population* control group is worked out in just the same way: odds of anaemia in cases is 44 divided by 102 = 0.43; odds of anaemia in population controls is 17 divided by 130 = 0.13; odds ratio is 0.43 divided by 0.13 = 3.3.

What does the odds ratio tell us? Researchers use the odds ratio not because it conveys meaning to the reader but because it has mathematical properties that we can only touch on here. As an expression of the comparison between the two kinds of chance, it is not easy to interpret. It cannot readily be 'translated' into anything more meaningful; it is purely the fraction formed by dividing the odds of being anaemic in one group by the odds in the other. If you have trouble figuring out what it tells you, don't worry: no one else can do any better than you. The nearest we can get to a common-sense way of expressing this result is to conclude that there is about three times the odds of being anaemic if you had a febrile seizure compared with if you didn't have a seizure. Just as with the risk ratio, remember that if the odds ratio is 1, then the odds is the same in each group being compared.

One key property of the odds ratio (and one of the reasons why researchers employ such an uninviting measure) can be illustrated from the table in Figure 18.2. Concentrate on the comparison of cases with hospital controls: we are going to rework the calculations in a different direction. In this study, if a child was anaemic, then the odds of him or her being in the case group (had a seizure) rather than in the hospital control group (didn't have a seizure) is 44 divided by 21 = 2.1. Similarly, if a child was not anaemic the odds of her or him being in the case group is 102 divided by 125 = 0.82. These odds can be compared in an odds ratio: 2.1 divided by 0.82 = 2.6. If you are sharp-eyed you will have spotted that this is the same odds ratio as the one we calculated previously, from a different direction.

We can now draw a new conclusion: that there is about three times the odds of getting a febrile convulsion if you're anaemic, compared with if you're not anaemic. This new conclusion is a much more useful one than the conclusion in the previous paragraph. After all, we don't want to conclude after the event that a child who had a convulsion is likely to have been anaemic; rather, we want to conclude that anaemia is a risky state that makes convulsions more likely (so we can do something about anaemic babies and toddlers and thereby prevent seizures).

When a condition is relatively uncommon (and most children don't have a febrile seizure, so it counts as an uncommon condition), the odds ratio is approximately the same as the risk ratio (we are not proving why here, but the straightforward proof can be found in most epidemiology books). This transferable property of odds ratios and risk ratios means that from the present study we can assert that small children in the catchment area of this Naples hospital have about three times the *risk* of getting a febrile convulsion if they are anaemic.

Of course the researchers could have carried out a cohort study instead and calculated the risk ratio directly – without all this jiggery-pokery. But because febrile convulsions are infrequent, a cohort study would have needed to include many thousands of children in order to come up with around 150 children who had sustained a seizure. The properties of the odds ratio enable researchers to carry out small, quick, cheap case–control studies (rather than large, lengthy and expensive cohort analytic studies) yet come up with clinically useful findings. Case–control studies almost always report their findings in terms of odds ratios.

CLINICAL TRIALS AND 'NUMBERS NEEDED TO TREAT'

Just about everyone finds it easier to comprehend risk ratios than odds ratios. Odds and odds ratios have other properties (not gone into here) that make them valuable in complex mathematics like multivariable analysis (Chapter 25) and meta-analysis (Chapter 26). Unfortunately this seems to have led many researchers to calculate and display their study findings as odds ratios even when they could have given us a risk ratio instead. Consequently, some clinicians – concerned that useful research output was being lost in a fog of incomprehensible numbers – have recently come up with what has become a popular way of making sense of some study findings. Where the results of a study come from a clinical trial of treatment or healthcare management, the *number needed to treat* (NNT) is a simple calculation and appeals to many as an intuitively straightforward way to get at the clinical meaning of the finding of a clinical trial.

As an example, researchers across three continents (though mainly in North America) collaborated in a large study to determine what dose of acetylsalicylic acid (aspirin) is the most beneficial to patients undergoing carotid artery surgery (aimed at preventing strokes). They found that fewer patients had a bad outcome (stroke, myocardial infarction or death) among the low-dose aspirin regimen than among those taking a high dose (Figure 18.3). For the analysis the researchers amalgamated the two lower dose regimens and the two higher dose regimens to end up with two (rather than four) comparison groups.

In their table you can see that for the various outcomes, at 30 days and 3 months, they have set out their findings as relative risks (risk ratios) – all falling at around 1.3. But in an attempt to make their findings easier for clinicians to apply in real situations, they have also calculated and displayed the number needed to treat derived from each of their comparisons. Figure 18.3 indicates how they have worked out the number needed to treat. For this calculation, instead of putting the two risks (one for each comparison group) into a ratio, they have subtracted them to generate a difference (sometimes called *absolute difference*) between the risks.

Looking at the top line of their table, notice that the reduction in risk due to the better of the two treatments (low-dose aspirin) is 7.0%−5.4% = 1.6%. Put another way, a reduction in risk of 1.6% means that of every 100 people treated with low-dose aspirin (rather than high-dose) 1.6 fewer will have a bad outcome (if you don't like 1.6 people, think of 16 people in a thousand – it's the same thing). It is a simple calculation then to say that if 100 treated with low-dose leads to 1.6 fewer bad outcomes, then 100/1.6 (about 61, allowing for some rounding in the arithmetic) people treated with low-dose will result in one less bad outcome. The general formula for the number needed to treat is that it is 100 divided by the percentage absolute risk reduction:

$$\text{Number needed to treat} = 100/\text{percentage absolute risk reduction}$$

This resulting value can be interpreted as follows: 'You would need to treat 61 patients scheduled for carotid endarterectomy with low-dose rather than high-dose aspirin in order to prevent one *extra* patient from experiencing the bad outcome (in this case stroke, heart attack or death).' Of course, this figure is only an estimate and it might have been displayed together with its confidence interval (not provided in the paper, but would be very wide). The number needed to treat is attractive to clinicians who may want to make judgements on the basis of the size of the effect found in a study.

Low-dose and high-dose acetylsalicylic acid for patients undergoing carotid endarterectomy: a randomised controlled trial

D Wayne Taylor, Henry J M Barnett, R Brian Haynes, Gary G Ferguson, David L Sackett, Kevin E Thorpe, Denis Simard, Frank L Silver, Vladimir Hachinski, G Patrick Clagett, R Barnes, J David Spence, for the ASA and Carotid Endarterectomy (ACE) Trial Collaborators*

Summary

Background Endarterectomy benefits certain patients with carotid stenosis, but benefits are lessened by perioperative surgical risk. Acetylsalicylic acid lowers the risk of stroke in patients who have experienced transient ischaemic attack and stroke. We investigated appropriate doses and the role of acetylsalicylic acid in patients undergoing carotid endarterectomy.

Methods In a randomised, double-blind, controlled trial, 2849 patients scheduled for endarterectomy were randomly assigned 81 mg (n=709), 325 mg (n=708), 650 mg (n=715), or 1300 mg (n=717) acetylsalicylic acid daily, started before surgery and continued for 3 months. We recorded occurrences of stroke, myocardial infarction, and death. We compared patients on the two higher doses of acetylsalicylic acid with patients on the two lower doses.

Number needed to treat (NNT) is applied usually to findings from trials and meta-analyses.

The comparison here is between low-dose (81 or 325 mg) and high-dose (650 or 1300 mg).

If you take away the risk of a bad outcome in the low-dose group (5.4%) from the risk in the high-dose group (7.0%) you get the difference in risks (1.6%).

Divide 100 by 1.6 and you find the NNT: around 61.

Event-defining failure	Event rate		Relative risk high/low dose (95% CI)	Absolute difference (% [SE])	p	NNT
	Low-dose ASA	High-dose ASA				
All patients						
30 days						
Number of patients	1395	1409	..	..	..	..
Any stroke, MI, or death	75 (5.4%)	99 (7.0%)	1.31 (0.98–1.75)	1.6 (0.9)	0.07	61
Any stroke or death	66 (4.7%)	86 (6.1%)	1.29 (0.94–1.76)	1.4 (0.9)	0.109	72
Ipsilateral stroke or death	58 (4.2%)	81 (5.7%)	1.38 (1.0–1.92)	1.6 (0.8)	0.052	62
3 months						
Number of patients	1395	1409	..	..	..	..
Any stroke, MI, or death	87 (6.2%)	118 (8.4%)	1.34 (1.03–1.75)	2.1 (1.0)	0.03	46
Any stroke or death	79 (5.7%)	100 (7.1%)	1.25 (0.94–1.67)	1.4 (0.9)	0.12	69
Ipsilateral stroke or death	68 (4.9%)	91 (6.5%)	1.32 (0.98–1.80)	1.6 (0.9)	0.07	63

Figure 4: **Failure rates at 30 days after endarterectomy**

FIGURE 18.3 Table from a clinical trial where the main findings are set out in terms of risk ratios together with numbers needed to treat

VI

Analysing the Data: Estimation and Hypothesis Testing

19

Confidence Intervals for Means, Proportions and Medians

You will remember from Chapter 8 that clinical researchers use *samples* to study aspects of 'groups of people', i.e. *populations*. What applies to the sample is taken to apply also to the population (always provided of course that the sample is truly representative of the population). The technical term for this process is *statistical inference*. For example, if the mean systolic blood pressure of a representative sample of men aged 45 to 65 is calculated to be 126.4 mmHg (this value being known as the *sample point estimate*), then we can *infer* that the mean systolic blood pressure of all of the men in the population is also 126.4 mmHg – *more or less*. The 'more or less' bit is crucially important, because no sample will be exactly identical to the sampled population.

To take account of this uncertainty, the researchers in the above example would have to qualify their estimate of the population mean systolic blood pressure, and give a value something like '126.4 ± 10.0 mmHg'. Don't worry where the value of ±10 mmHg for the 'more or less' bit came from for the moment, let's just say that it's easily calculated. In fact it's bad form to present this result in the ± format. Better is to express the estimate as:

$$(126.4 - 10.0) \text{ to } (126.4 + 10.0) \text{ mmHg}$$
$$\text{or} \qquad (116.4 \text{ to } 136.4) \text{ mmHg}$$

This way of expressing the result is known as a *confidence interval*. What it tells us is that the true mean systolic blood pressure of all such men in the sampled population is *likely* to be between 116.4 mmHg and 136.4 mmHg. You're already asking, 'How likely?' Conventionally, researchers want to be 95% confident that their estimate is correct. So an interval such as (116.4 to 136.4) mmHg would be called a *95% confidence interval estimate*, or just a 95% confidence interval (often abbreviated in papers to 95% CI). Statisticians say that a confidence interval represents *a plausible range of values* for the true (population) value.

The *width* of a confidence interval quoted in a paper also provides the reader with a way of assessing the *precision of the estimate*. Suppose, as an illustration of this point, that the 95% confidence interval for mean systolic blood pressure had been (86.4 to 176.4) mmHg. Since the confidence interval provides us with a range of values within which we are most likely to find the true population mean systolic blood pressure, then an interval as wide as this one is of very little help – the value could be anywhere between 86.4 mmHg and 176.4 mmHg! The original interval of (116.4 to 136.4) mmHg enables us to form a much more precise estimate of the true population mean.

In general, when estimating a particular population value, the larger the sample, the narrower and thus more precise is the confidence interval. When you are examining confidence intervals in a paper, you need to look out for confidence intervals which are too wide to be of much help, even though they may be statistically significant.

Clinical papers, if they have any statistical content at all, will often include confidence intervals for one or more population values. When you are reading such a paper you need to be able to tell which population value is being estimated and what *level of confidence* the authors have used (usually 95%, but sometimes 99%, and on rare occasions 90%). Authors should present a confidence interval with the word

Understanding Clinical Papers Second Edition   David Bowers, Allan House, David Owens
© 2006 John Wiley & Sons, Ltd

'to' in the middle, as in (116.4 *to* 136.4) mmHg, rather than with a hyphen, since this avoids possible confusion when one or both of the values in the confidence interval have a minus sign (see Chapter 28). It is not helpful to separate the values by a comma, as in (116.4, 136.4) mmHg. The $\pm$ form is lazy and inconsiderate, you have to do the arithmetic yourself!

CONFIDENCE INTERVALS FOR DIFFERENCES IN MEANS

Researchers frequently use confidence intervals to determine whether or not there is a significant *difference* between two population values, for example, between the mean systolic blood pressure of males and females. Obviously if the two means *are* the same, then the difference between them will be zero. We could therefore, very easily, use an appropriate computer program (SPSS, Minitab, Stata, etc.) to provide an estimate of the difference between these two population means, along with a 95% confidence interval.

Suppose we did this and got a 95% CI of (4.5 to 9.1) mmHg. In other words, we can be 95% confident that the true difference between the two population mean systolic blood pressures is between 4.5 mmHg and 9.1 mmHg. (Note that we might just as easily have got the result (-9.1 to -4.5) mmHg. Which result you get depends on the order in which you enter the variables into the computer program.) Crucially, this interval *does not include 0*, so we can be 95% certain that the difference between the two population means is not zero. Put another way, the interval from 4.5 mmHg to 9.1 mmHg represents a *plausible range of values* for the true difference between the population means.

However, suppose the interval was (-2.4 to 3.7) mmHg. This implies that the difference in the population values could be anywhere between -2.4 mmHg and 3.7 mmHg. Crucially, since this interval now *includes 0*, we would have to conclude that there may very well be no difference between the mean systolic blood pressures of the males and females in the population. As we noted above, confidence intervals can be calculated for many different population parameters (or the differences between them). In this chapter we are going to concentrate on the three most commonly seen in clinical papers: the mean, the proportion, and the median.

In the next study the authors were investigating differences in mean bone mineral densities between depressed and 'normal' women. The second and third columns of Figure 19.1 show the sample mean bone mineral densities at six sites for both groups of women. The fourth column contains estimates of the *differences* in mean bone densities along with their 95% confidence intervals (ignore the 'SD from expected peak' rows).

Thus, at the lumbar spine the mean bone mineral density for the depressed women was 1.00 g/cm (SD = 0.15 g/cm^2), for the non-depressed women it was 1.07 g/cm^2 (SD = 0.09 g/cm^2). The difference in sample means is thus 0.08 g/cm^2 (1.07 minus 1.00, allowing for rounding errors). So the sample mean bone density at the lumbar spine is 0.08 g/cm^2 more dense in the normal women than in the depressed women. The 95% confidence interval for the difference in means, (0.02 to 0.14), provides a plausible range for the *true* difference. This interval *does not contain 0*, so we can be 95% confident that there *is* a significant difference in mean bone mineral density at the lumbar spine between the two groups of women. In other words a *plausible range of values for the true difference* is that it lies somewhere between 0.02 and 0.14 g/cm^2.

The crucial question you need to ask is thus: *Does the confidence interval for the difference include zero?* If it does, then there may very well be *no* difference in the two population values. If it does not, then there probably is a difference. Moreover, the true difference is likely to be somewhere in the quoted interval.

The other confidence intervals show that all differences in mean bone density are significant (normal women have denser bones than depressed women at all sites) *except* for the radius bone. Here the interval is from -0.01 g/cm^2 to 0.04 g/cm^2, which *does* include zero. Since zero is a possible value, it can't be ruled out as being the true value.

BONE MINERAL DENSITY IN WOMEN WITH DEPRESSION

DAVID MICHELSON, M.D., CONSTANTINE STRATAKIS, M.D., PHD., LAUREN HILL, B.S., JAMES REYNOLDS, M.D., ELISE GALLIVEN, B.S., GEORGE CHROUSOS, M.D., AND PHILIP GOLD M.D.

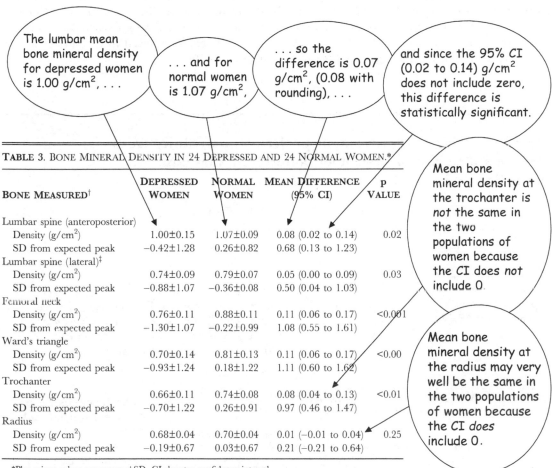

The lumbar mean bone mineral density for depressed women is 1.00 g/cm², . . .

. . . and for normal women is 1.07 g/cm²,

. . . so the difference is 0.07 g/cm², (0.08 with rounding), . . .

and since the 95% CI (0.02 to 0.14) g/cm² does not include zero, this difference is statistically significant.

Mean bone mineral density at the trochanter is not the same in the two populations of women because the CI does not include 0.

Mean bone mineral density at the radius may very well be the same in the two populations of women because the CI does include 0.

TABLE 3. BONE MINERAL DENSITY IN 24 DEPRESSED AND 24 NORMAL WOMEN.*

BONE MEASURED[†]	DEPRESSED WOMEN	NORMAL WOMEN	MEAN DIFFERENCE (95% CI)	p VALUE
Lumbar spine (anteroposterior)				
Density (g/cm²)	1.00±0.15	1.07±0.09	0.08 (0.02 to 0.14)	0.02
SD from expected peak	−0.42±1.28	0.26±0.82	0.68 (0.13 to 1.23)	
Lumbar spine (lateral)[‡]				
Density (g/cm²)	0.74±0.09	0.79±0.07	0.05 (0.00 to 0.09)	0.03
SD from expected peak	−0.88±1.07	−0.36±0.08	0.50 (0.04 to 1.03)	
Femoral neck				
Density (g/cm²)	0.76±0.11	0.88±0.11	0.11 (0.06 to 0.17)	<0.001
SD from expected peak	−1.30±1.07	−0.22±0.99	1.08 (0.55 to 1.61)	
Ward's triangle				
Density (g/cm²)	0.70±0.14	0.81±0.13	0.11 (0.06 to 0.17)	<0.00
SD from expected peak	−0.93±1.24	0.18±1.22	1.11 (0.60 to 1.62)	
Trochanter				
Density (g/cm²)	0.66±0.11	0.74±0.08	0.08 (0.04 to 0.13)	<0.01
SD from expected peak	−0.70±1.22	0.26±0.91	0.97 (0.46 to 1.47)	
Radius				
Density (g/cm²)	0.68±0.04	0.70±0.04	0.01 (−0.01 to 0.04)	0.25
SD from expected peak	−0.19±0.67	0.03±0.67	0.21 (−0.21 to 0.64)	

*Plus-minus values are means ±SD. CI denotes confidence interval.

[†]Values for "SD from expected peak" are the numbers of standard deviations from the expected peak density derived from a population-based study of normal white women.[3]

[‡]This measurement was made in 23 depressed women and 23 normal women.

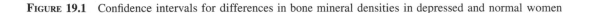

FIGURE 19.1 Confidence intervals for differences in bone mineral densities in depressed and normal women

CONFIDENCE INTERVALS FOR DIFFERENCES IN PROPORTIONS

In the next example the authors investigated the effects of improving nutrition on respiratory infections and diarrhoeal disease in Vietnamese preschool children. They compared the incidence and severity of these two illnesses in the children in two communes, one which had benefited from an Australian nutrition project from 1991 to the end of 1993, the other which had received no such input. The children were surveyed every three months from March 1992 until April 1993, so there were five data collection periods. Figure 19.2 shows 95% confidence intervals for the difference in the *proportion* of children in the two communes who suffered diarrhoeal disease in the two-week period prior to each data collection period. The results indicate that levels of diarrhoea were significantly reduced in the later collection periods, as the benefits of the nutritional programme began to be felt.

Effect of nutrition improvement project on morbidity from infectious diseases in preschool children in Vietnam: comparison with control commune

R M English, J C Badcock, Tu Giay, Tu Ngu, A-M Waters, S A Bennett

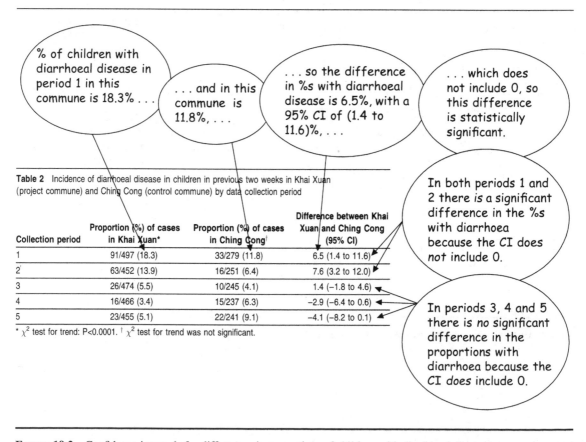

% of children with diarrhoeal disease in period 1 in this commune is 18.3% . . .

. . . and in this commune is 11.8%, . . .

. . . so the difference in %s with diarrhoeal disease is 6.5%, with a 95% CI of (1.4 to 11.6)%, . . .

. . . which does not include 0, so this difference is statistically significant.

Table 2 Incidence of diarrhoeal disease in children in previous two weeks in Khai Xuan (project commune) and Ching Cong (control commune) by data collection period

In both periods 1 and 2 there *is* a significant difference in the %s with diarrhoea because the CI does *not* include 0.

Collection period	Proportion (%) of cases in Khai Xuan*	Proportion (%) of cases in Ching Cong[†]	Difference between Khai Xuan and Ching Cong (95% CI)
1	91/497 (18.3)	33/279 (11.8)	6.5 (1.4 to 11.6)
2	63/452 (13.9)	16/251 (6.4)	7.6 (3.2 to 12.0)
3	26/474 (5.5)	10/245 (4.1)	1.4 (−1.8 to 4.6)
4	16/466 (3.4)	15/237 (6.3)	−2.9 (−6.4 to 0.6)
5	23/455 (5.1)	22/241 (9.1)	−4.1 (−8.2 to 0.1)

* χ^2 test for trend: P<0.0001. [†] χ^2 test for trend was not significant.

In periods 3, 4 and 5 there is *no significant* difference in the proportions with diarrhoea because the CI *does* include 0.

FIGURE 19.2 Confidence intervals for differences in proportions of children with diarrhoeal disease in two communes

CONFIDENCE INTERVALS FOR DIFFERENCES IN MEDIANS

Let's return to the study first encountered in Figure 12.2 on the efficacy of bupivacaine given before amputation for the relief of post-amputation stump pain. Patient pre-amputation pain was measured in both the treatment and control groups. The median pain levels for the two groups are shown in Figure 19.3, along with 95% confidence intervals for differences in median pain levels between the two groups.

We can see that the differences in median pain levels between the treatment and control (placebo) groups are significant at all the time points since none of the confidence intervals includes zero. For example, after the epidural bolus (of either bupivacaine or saline), the median pain levels were 0 and 38 respectively. Thus the difference was 38 and the 95% confidence interval for the true difference was (24 to 43) which does not include 0. So a plausible range for the true difference in the medians is somewhere between 24 and 43.

Confidence intervals are used in many contexts of which the three above are among the most widely encountered. If you are trying to understand a confidence interval for the true value of the *difference* in some measure between two groups, then the general rule is as follows:

If the confidence interval for the difference contains 0, you can be 95% confident (or 99%, or whatever confidence level is stated) that there is no statistically significant difference between the groups in terms of the measure in question. If the interval does not contain 0, then there is a statistically significant difference. You can also be 95% confident that the confidence interval contains the true value of any difference in the measures.

Randomised trial of epidural bupivacaine and morphine in prevention of stump and phantom pain lower-limb amputation

Lone Nikolajsen, Susanne Ilkjaer, Jørgen H Christensen, Karsten Krøner, Troels S Jensen

	Median (IQR) pain		
	Blockade group (n=27)	Control group (n=29)	95% CI for difference (p)
After epidural bolus	0 (0–0)	38 (17–67)	24 to 43 (p<0.0001)
After continuous epidural infusion	0 (0–0)	31 (20–51)	24 to 43 (p<0.0001)
After epidural bolus in operating theatre	0 (0–0)	35 (16–64)	19 to 42 (p<0.0001)

Pain assessed by visual analogue scale (0–100 mm).

Table 2: **Intensity of preamputation pain during treatment with bupivacaine and morphine (blockade group) or saline (control group)**

A plausible range of values for the true difference in median pain levels after the epidural bolus is from 24 to 43 . . .

. . . and there is a *significant* difference in median pain levels between the two groups at each stage, because *none* of the CIs includes 0.

FIGURE 19.3   Confidence intervals for differences in median preoperative pain levels in the stump pain study

CONFIDENCE INTERVALS FOR A SINGLE POPULATION VALUE

Although a lot of papers contain confidence intervals for differences between two population values, they may also include confidence intervals for a *single* population value. Figure 19.4 shows the confidence intervals for the population mean scores on the objective structured clinical examinations (OSCE) of two groups of medical students, taught for their first five weeks of blocks 1 and 2, either in general practice or in hospital (ignore the last column for now). The values P and Q in the table refer to two parallel nine-station OSCEs.

For example, the students in general practice, following route P, and in block P1, had a mean OSCE score of 37.8 marks in the History-taking strand, with a 95% CI of (36.2 to 39.4). From this result we can be 95% confident that the mean OSCE score of *all* the students in the population for whom this sample is representative will have a mean OSCE score somewhere between 36.2 and 39.4 marks.

Similar students in a hospital setting had a higher mean OSCE score of 39.9 marks, with a 95% CI of (38.2 to 41.6) marks. As it happens, the authors chose to compare these two mean scores using a hypothesis test (we'll come to those in Chapter 21), but they could have calculated confidence intervals

Can students learn clinical method in general practice? A randomised crossover trial based on objective structured clinical examinations

Elizabeth Murray, Brian Jolly, Michael Modell

Table 1 Comparison of mean scores on objective structured clinical examinations (OSCE) of students taught for their first five weeks of blocks 1 and 2 either in general practice or in hospital

Skill domain	OSCE and block	Mean score (95% CI) General practice	Mean score (95% CI) Hospital	p value
History taking (max score 60)	P1	37.8 (36.2 to 39.4)	39.9 (38.2 to 41.6)	NS
	Q2	38.4 (36.4 to 40.4)	36.6 (34.3 to 39)	NS
Physical examination (max score 60)	P1	35.9 (33.0 to 38.8)	36.6 (33.3 to 40.0)	NS
	Q2	45.0 (41.8 to 48.2)	41.7 (39.9 to 43.5)	NS
Communication skills (max score 20)	P1	12.0 (10.8 to 13.2)	12.4 (11.7 to 13.2)	NS
	Q2	10.2 (9.4 to 11.0)	10.1 (9.3 to 10.9)	NS
Data interpretation (max score 40)	P1	24.4 (23.0 to 25.8)	26.9 (25.4 to 28.3)	0.02
	Q2	21.0 (19.4 to 22.6)	17.4 (15.5 to 19.4)	0.007
Total score (max score 180)	P1	110.1 (106.1 to 114.1)	115.9 (111.7 to 120)	NS
	Q2	114.6 (109.2 to 120.1)	105.9 (101.3 to 110.6)	0.02

Students who took OSCE P1 (n=56) had had a four week introductory course before their medical attachment, students who took OSCE Q2 (n=54) had had the four week introductory course plus 10 weeks of a surgical attachment.

The true mean score of these general practice students is between 36.2% and 39.4%, . . .

. . . while for these hospital students it's between 38.2% and 41.6%. The fact that the intervals overlap tells us that there is probably no difference between the mean scores of the two groups.

FIGURE 19.4 95% confidence intervals for mean OSCE scores of two groups of medical students

for the *difference* in means and interpreted them appropriately (as we saw above). Notice that although the table conveys quite clearly which confidence intervals have been calculated, it is not so easy to determine the sample size of the subgroups involved in each case.

As well as being used for *single* means, medians and proportions, confidence intervals are also frequently quoted for things like: prevalences; rates (incidence rates, mortality rates, etc.); counts; diagnostic measures (like sensitivity, specificity); and many other measures, a lot of which we will encounter in the following chapter. Of course, when confidence intervals are calculated for single measures, rather than for the *difference* in measures, we are not as much concerned with knowing whether the confidence interval includes 0, as with viewing the interval as a measure of the precision of our estimate, and offering us a plausible range of values for the true (population) value.

As a final example, Figure 19.5 is taken from a cross-sectional study to measure, first, the prevalence of genital chlamydia among British women, and second, the screening performance of a relatively new test for the condition, the ligase chain reaction test. This will be compared to an enzyme immunoassay (taken as the gold standard).

Figure 19.5 shows values for the prevalence, and for the four main diagnostic measures, for both screening procedures applied to 765 women. We see that the true prevalence of genital chlamydia as measured by the enzyme immunoassay is most probably somewhere between 0.8% and 2.7% (single best guess, 1.6%), whereas using the ligase chain reaction it's most probably between 1.5% and 3.9% (single best guess, 2.5%). If the true prevalence was zero (i.e. no British woman had this disease), then it's possible that the confidence interval could include 0. However, in most practical circumstances the 'includes 0' criterion is of secondary importance. As for the four diagnostic measures, only sensitivity shows any noticeable difference in the performance of the two screening methods.

To sum up, if you are reading a paper that contains confidence intervals, you should easily be able to tell what true value (for example, the true difference between two means) the confidence interval is calculated for, what level of confidence has been used, and if subgroups are being analysed, what the sample size is in each case.

There is another important class of measures for which confidence intervals are commonly quoted, that of *ratios*. In the next chapter we will see how the interpretation of the confidence interval for a ratio is markedly different.

Comparison of two methods of screening for genital chlamydial infection in women attending in general practice: cross sectional survey

Lucia Grun, Julia Tassano-Smith, Caroline Carder, Anne M Johnson, Angela Robinson, Elizabeth Murray, Judith Stephenson, Andrew Haines, Andrew Copas, Geoffrey Ridgway

Table 1 Comparison of performance of ligase chain reaction testing on urine with that of enzyme immunoassay of endocervical specimens in 765 women aged 18–35

| | Lipase chain reaction | | Enzyme immunoassay | |
	No of women	% (95% CI)	No of women	% (95% CI)
Prevalence	19/765	2.5 (1.5 to 3.9)	12/765	1.6 (0.8 to 2.7)
Sensitivity	18/20	90 (68 to 99)	12/20	60 (36 to 81)
Specificity	744/745	99.9 (99.2 to 100)	745/745	100 (99.5 to 100)
Predictive value of positive result	18/19	95 (74 to 100)	12/12	100 (74 to 100)
Predictive value of negative result	744/746	99.7 (99 to 100)	745/753	98.9 (97.9 to 99.5)

> Prevalence of the infection using the ligase chain reaction test is 2.5%, but the true value could be anywhere between 1.5% and 3.9%.

> With the enzyme immunoassay test, prevalence is only 1.6%, but the true value could be anywhere between 0.8% and 2.7%.

FIGURE 19.5 Table of prevalence and four diagnostic measures (with 95% CIs) comparing immunoassay and ligase chain reaction for screening for genital chlamydia

Confidence Intervals for Ratios

You will recall the discussion in Chapters 17 and 18 on risk and risk ratios (often called *relative risk*) and odds and odds ratios. Clinical researchers need to calculate confidence intervals for the true (population) values of these ratios just as much as they do for the measures discussed in Chapter 19. When you read papers which contain the results of such calculations, you still need to able to tell which ratio the confidence interval applies to, what level of confidence has been used, and which sample the confidence interval has been based on.

However, there is an important difference in the way confidence intervals for ratios, such as the odds ratio and risk ratio, are interpreted. In Chapter 19 we saw that if a confidence interval includes zero, then we could reasonably assume no statistically significant difference between the population measures. The notable exception to this rule is the interpretation of CIs for *ratios*, such as the *odds ratio*, *risk ratio* and *hazard ratio*. Risk ratios are commonly associated with *cohort* studies, odds ratios with *case–control* studies, and hazard ratios with *survival analysis*, discussed further in Chapter 27.

In clinical papers you will more often see odds ratios than risk ratios. One reason for this is the ease with which they can be calculated using logistic regression methods – the delights of which you will encounter in Chapter 25. In practice, we can use the odds ratio as a proxy for the risk ratio *provided* that the condition is rare (a prevalence of less than 10%, say) and interpret both measures to mean much the same thing (see Chapter 18). For example, authors quite often calculate odds ratios in a case–control study (using logistic regression) and then interpret them using terms like 'risk', and 'risk factor'.

However, it is worth bearing in mind that when odds ratios are quoted for high-prevalence conditions or outcomes, they may not be similar to the corresponding risk ratios. This is something you need to look out for when you read a paper containing such measures. You need to able to tell what the prevalence of the condition or outcome in question is, especially if the authors are using the odds ratio as a proxy for the risk ratio. In case–control and cohort studies, but not necessarily in clinical trials, the prevalence will usually be low enough for the equivalence between odds and risk ratios to be acceptable.

CONFIDENCE INTERVALS FOR ODDS RATIOS

Let's get back to the different way in which confidence intervals for ratios like the odds ratio are interpreted. An example given at the end of Chapter 17 reported an odds ratio of 1.06 for ischaemic heart disease (IHD) among men with *H. pylori* compared with men without *H. pylori*. In other words, men with *H. pylori* have 1.06 times the odds of IHD than men without. In other words, compared to men without *H. pylori* infection, 6% more men with *H. pylori* infection have ischaemic heart disease.

What if the odds ratio had been equal to 1? This would imply that the odds for ischaemic heart disease were *evenly* matched between the two groups; that is the presence or absence of *H. pylori* makes no *significant difference* to the odds of having IHD. Going further, imagine now that the odds ratio had been *less than* 1, for example, 0.75. This would imply that having *H. pylori* in some way *protects* against

Understanding Clinical Papers Second Edition   David Bowers, Allan House, David Owens
© 2006 John Wiley & Sons, Ltd

IHD! To sum up, when you want to assess the nature of a 'risk' factor from a confidence interval for a ratio quoted in a paper, you need to ask the following question:

Is the odds ratio greater than 1? If so, the factor concerned is a possible risk; if less than 1, it's a possible 'benefit'. If the odds ratio equals 1, the factor makes no difference either way.

We use the word 'possible' here because we still have to decide on statistical significance, since, as ever, odds ratios calculated from samples are only estimates of the true (population) values. In this respect, you need to know whether the interval *contains 1 or not* in contrast to whether or not it contains 0 for many of the examples in Chapter 19. The reason is of course that if two numbers are the same and you subtract them (to find the difference) you get 0, whereas if you divide them (to form the ratio) the result is 1.

If a 95% confidence interval for an odds ratio *does* contain 1, then we can be 95% confident that the condition or risk factor involved is *not* significant, either as a risk or a benefit. On the other hand, if the confidence interval *does not contain 1*, we can be 95% confident that the condition *is* a significant risk or benefit, and interpret its exact status using the rule above.

So when you look at the confidence interval for an odds ratio you want to know if it contains 1. If it does, the factor concerned plays no significant role; if it doesn't, the factor is a significant risk (or benefit). Note that, as was the case for the confidence intervals discussed in Chapter 19, the width of the interval is also a measure of the precision of the estimate. Wider intervals are less precise and therefore less useful. Incidentally, the risk factor *H. pylori* is not a significant risk factor for ischaemic heart disease since the 95% confidence interval of (0.86 to 1.31) quoted in Chapter 17 includes 1.

Have a look now at Figure 20.1 which reports odds ratios and their 95% CIs from a study into a number of possible risk factors for genital chlamydia. The 890 subjects were women attending several general practices in London between 1994 and 1996, and diagnosed with genital chlamydia. One of the risk factors being examined is number of sexual partners in the past year. In the main body of the text, the authors provide the desired information on the prevalence of genital chlamydia. In the sample it was calculated to be 2.6% with a 95% CI of (1.6% to 3.6%), figures compatible with an assumption of low prevalence, thus assuring approximate equivalence of the odds ratio and risk ratio measures.

Figure 20.1 shows that compared with women with either no partner or 1 partner (defined as the *referent* group with an odds ratio of 1), women with two or more partners had an odds ratio for genital chlamydia of 2.83, i.e. these women had nearly three times the odds of having the disease. The 95% CI is given as (1.19 to 7.18) and since this does not include 1, we can reasonably assume that having two or more partners *is* a statistically significant risk factor. We can be 95% confident that the *true* value for the odds ratio among *all* similar women lies somewhere between 1.19 and 7.18. Notice, by the way, that the value for the odds ratio does not sit in the middle of its confidence interval, unlike the case with the confidence intervals for means, proportions, counts, and their differences.

Another potential risk factor considered was marital status. The referent group here is defined as single women. Compared with these, married women in the sample had an odds ratio of 0.19. At first sight this suggests that being married is therefore a protective factor against genital chlamydia. Married women have only about a fifth (1/0.19) the odds of contracting the disease compared with single women. However, in this case the 95% confidence interval, given as (0.02 to 1.45), *includes* the value 1, so we can conclude from this result that marital status, is *not* a statistically significant factor in the occurrence of genital chlamydia. Bear in mind though that a larger sample might have produced a narrower, more precise confidence interval, even possibly one that did not contain 1.

Apart from number of partners in the past year, the only other statistically significant risk factor was age. In particular, women aged 20 or less had over eight times the odds of having genital chlamydia

Comparison of two methods of screening for genital chlamydial infection in women attending in general practice: cross sectional survey

Lucia Grun, Julia Tassano-Smith, Caroline Carder, Anne M Johnson, Angela Robinson, Elizabeth Murray, Judith Stephenson, Andrew Haines, Andrew Copas, Geoffrey Ridgway

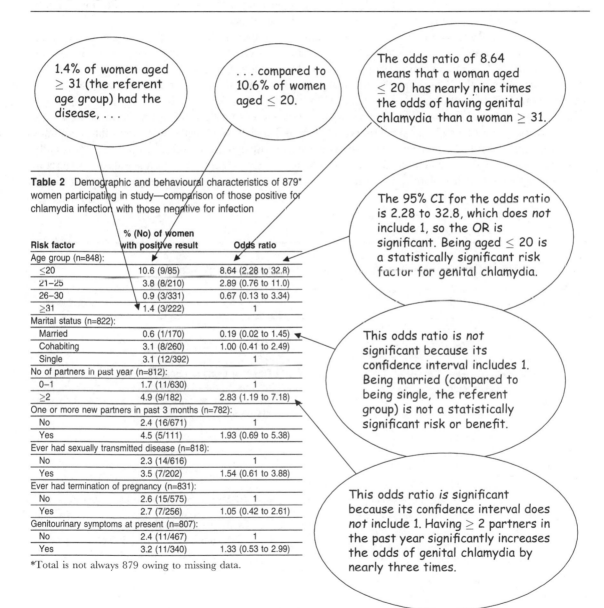

Table 2 Demographic and behavioural characteristics of 879* women participating in study—comparison of those positive for chlamydia infection with those negative for infection

Risk factor	% (No) of women with positive result	Odds ratio
Age group (n=848):		
≤20	10.6 (9/85)	8.64 (2.28 to 32.8)
21–25	3.8 (8/210)	2.89 (0.76 to 11.0)
26–30	0.9 (3/331)	0.67 (0.13 to 3.34)
≥31	1.4 (3/222)	1
Marital status (n=822):		
Married	0.6 (1/170)	0.19 (0.02 to 1.45)
Cohabiting	3.1 (8/260)	1.00 (0.41 to 2.49)
Single	3.1 (12/392)	1
No of partners in past year (n=812):		
0–1	1.7 (11/630)	1
≥2	4.9 (9/182)	2.83 (1.19 to 7.18)
One or more new partners in past 3 months (n=782):		
No	2.4 (16/671)	1
Yes	4.5 (5/111)	1.93 (0.69 to 5.38)
Ever had sexually transmitted disease (n=818):		
No	2.3 (14/616)	1
Yes	3.5 (7/202)	1.54 (0.61 to 3.88)
Ever had termination of pregnancy (n=831):		
No	2.6 (15/575)	1
Yes	2.7 (7/256)	1.05 (0.42 to 2.61)
Genitourinary symptoms at present (n=807):		
No	2.4 (11/467)	1
Yes	3.2 (11/340)	1.33 (0.53 to 2.99)

*Total is not always 879 owing to missing data.

1.4% of women aged ≥ 31 (the referent age group) had the disease, . . .

. . . compared to 10.6% of women aged ≤ 20.

The odds ratio of 8.64 means that a woman aged ≤ 20 has nearly nine times the odds of having genital chlamydia than a woman ≥ 31.

The 95% CI for the odds ratio is 2.28 to 32.8, which does not include 1, so the OR is significant. Being aged ≤ 20 is a statistically significant risk factor for genital chlamydia.

This odds ratio is not significant because its confidence interval includes 1. Being married (compared to being single, the referent group) is not a statistically significant risk or benefit.

This odds ratio is significant because its confidence interval does not include 1. Having ≥ 2 partners in the past year significantly increases the odds of genital chlamydia by nearly three times.

FIGURE 20.1   Odds ratios for risk factors for genital chlamydia

than women aged 31 and over, the 95% CI being reported as (2.28 to 32.8), which of course does not include 1.

CONFIDENCE INTERVALS FOR RISK RATIOS

We can interpret confidence intervals for risk ratios (relative risk) in just the same way as for odds ratios. If the confidence interval includes 1, then there is no statistically significant risk associated with the factor involved. If the confidence interval does not contain 1, then the risk ratio is significant – if less than 1 it is 'beneficial', if greater than 1 there is an adverse effect.

In the following study (see Figure 20.2) into health inequalities in the children of single mothers, the authors produced a table of relative risks (i.e. risk ratios) for child mortality by age and social group, along with the 95% confidence intervals. There is clear evidence that single mothers are most often classified as being in the 'Unoccupied' group, and it was the risk of child mortality in this group which was of interest to the authors.

In the figure, Social Groups I and II are taken as the referent group (with a risk ratio of 1), so the relative risks in the other groups are relative to Groups I and II. The last row of the table combines Groups IV and V with the Unoccupied group. The results show that all the relative risks are statistically significant since none of the confidence intervals contain 1. For example, children aged 10–15 years in the Unoccupied group had a risk of dying in childhood just over four times that of similarly aged

Health inequalities: new concerns about the children of single mothers

Ken Judge, Michaela Benzeval

	Age bands		
Social group	1–4 Years	5–9 Years	10–15 Years
I and II	1.00	1.00	1.00
	(0.83 to 1.21)	(0.80 to 1.25)	(0.84 to 1.20)
IV and V	2.08*	1.71*	1.37
	(1.75 to 2.49)	(1.39 to 2.12)	(1.14 to 1.64)
"Unoccupied"	2.58*	2.56*	4.14*
	(2.07 to 3.22)	(1.98 to 3.30)	(3.43 to 4.99)
IV, V and unoccupied	2.21*	1.93*	1.98*
	(1.88 to 2.61)	(1.59 to 2.35)	(1.69 to 2.32)

*$p < 0.05$.

Annotations:

The risk factor is membership of one of these four social groups.

Referent group (Social groups I and II) with risk ratio = 1 of dying in childhood.

10-15 year olds in the Unoccupied group have over four times the risk of death of childhood compared to 10-15 year olds in the Social Groups I and II. The CI does not include 1, so the risk is significant

FIGURE 20.2   Risk ratios for childhood mortality by social group

children in Social Groups I and II, with a 95% CI of (3.43 to 4.99). Notice the asterisks in the table referring to 'p'. We will consider this notation further in Chapter 21.

CONFIDENCE INTERVALS FOR HAZARD RATIOS

Odds ratios and risk ratios are the ratios you will perhaps see most frequently in the literature, but the *hazard ratio* (HR) is also important. The interpretation of confidence intervals for hazard ratios is similar to that for odds and risk ratios. If the interval contains 1, the factor is not a statistically significant risk. If it does not contain 1, the factor is a statistically significant risk. Values greater than 1 indicate that the factor increases the risk of death (or the specified clinical outcome), values less than 1 indicate that the factor decreases this risk. We will discuss the hazard ratio in more detail in the context of survival analysis later in the book when we introduce proportional hazards regression.

In addition to odds, risk and hazard ratios, clinical research papers will contain references to other ratios and their confidence intervals (for example, confidence intervals for the ratio of two population means is occasionally to be seen). Whatever the ratio, the rule described in this section, as to whether or not the confidence interval includes 1, still applies.

In Chapters 19 and 20 you have seen how confidence intervals can be helpful in the analysis of research results. In Chapter 21 we will discuss hypothesis testing, which offers an alternative approach, and examine the close relationship between confidence intervals and hypothesis tests.

21

Testing Hypotheses – the *p*-Value

As you will recall from Chapter 3, researchers usually start with a research objective or question. We have seen examples of this already: 'To find out if the bone mineral density of depressed and non-depressed women is different'; 'To investigate whether the number of sexual partners is a risk factor for genital chlamydia'; 'To see whether a telephone helpline can be effective in promoting smoking cessation'.

In Chapters 19 and 20 we saw that one way authors can answer such research questions is to calculate an appropriate confidence interval – for example, for the difference in mean bone mineral density, or for the odds ratio for number of sexual partners. An alternative approach sometimes used is that of *hypothesis testing*. We noted in Chapter 3 that the research objective is often expressed in the form of a null hypothesis (although not often explicitly). It is this *null hypothesis* which the researcher tests. For example:

Null hypothesis: There is *no difference* in bone density between depressed and non-depressed women.
Null hypothesis: The number of sexual partners is *not* a risk factor for genital chlamydia.

Conceptually, the hypothesis testing idea is not difficult. Researchers take a representative sample, examine the sample data for evidence *against* the null hypothesis, then decide whether this is strong enough for the null hypothesis to be *rejected*. How then do researchers decide what constitutes strong enough evidence? Since the evidence they use is a probability, a few words on probability seem appropriate.

A FEW WORDS ON PROBABILITY

The probability of any event can vary from 0 (meaning it cannot happen – like getting a total of 13 from rolling two dice), to 1 (it is certain to happen – like getting a number from 1 to 6 when one dice is rolled). The closer the probability is to 0, the less likely the event is to happen; the closer to 1 the more likely. If the probability equals 0.5, i.e. 1 in 2, then the event is as likely to happen as not.

If two events are *independent* then the probability of one event occurring is in no way related to the probability of the other event occurring. So for example, if we toss a coin twice and get a head with the first toss (the probability of which is 0.5), then the probability of a head on the second toss is also 0.5, because the two events are independent. The probability of getting two heads in succession is the product of the separate probabilities, i.e. $0.5 \times 0.5 = 0.25$, or 1 in 4. This multiplication rule can be extended to any number of independent events. Probability theory is a huge subject but that's all we need here.

ASSESSING THE EVIDENCE AGAINST THE NULL HYPOTHESIS – THE *p*-VALUE

The idea of the *p*-value is best illustrated with an example. Suppose you are a practice nurse and have invited all patients aged 65 or over to come for a pneumococcal vaccination. Your null hypothesis (usually denoted H_0), is that about equal numbers of males and females will attend. That is:

H_0: Equal numbers of males and females will come for their pneumococcal jab

---

Understanding Clinical Papers Second Edition   David Bowers, Allan House, David Owens
© 2006 John Wiley & Sons, Ltd

This hypothesis relates of course to the numbers attending in the *population* of over-65s. This population may be all over-65s in the practice, or across the city, or in the country. It depends which population you believe you sample is representative of.

You need some evidence to decide whether your null hypothesis can be sustained or rejected. The gender of the next 100 patients seems reasonable. If you get 48 males (and 52 females), you'll almost certainly *not* reject H_0. This outcome seems *quite probable* if the hypothesis of equal numbers is true. It offers scant evidence against the 50:50 hypothesis. (Remember that even if H_0 is true you are extremely unlikely to get 50 males and 50 females because of sampling variability.)

Suppose you get 10 males and 90 females. This outcome is *highly improbable*, and so offers very strong evidence *against* H_0. You are certain to *reject* H_0. However, suppose you get 40 males and 60 females. The decision now is much harder. How probable is this outcome if H_0 is true? Does this outcome offer strong enough evidence against H_0 or not? Obviously you need a systematic way of deciding. This where the *p*-value comes in. We can define the *p*-value as follows:

> the p-value is the probability of getting the outcome you get, or one more extreme, if H_0 is true.

So the *p*-value for the outcome 40 males is the probability of getting 40 males or 39 males or 38 or 37, down to 1 male or 0 males.[*] The critical probability is conventionally set at 0.05 (occasionally 0.01, rarely anything else). So if the *p*-value is <0.05, this is taken to offer strong evidence against H_0. Such an outcome is so improbable if H_0 is true that we are obliged to conclude that H_0 is probably not true, and we thus reject it.

One of the things you need to be able to tell, therefore, when reading through the results of a hypothesis test is what significance level the authors have used for their tests (usually 0.05, but sometimes 0.01). Furthermore, authors should report *p*-values clearly and in full (three significant decimal places is enough). For example, '*p*-value = 0.025' or 'a *p*-value of 0.155' or whatever, but not '*p*-value <0.05, or <0.01, or >0.05', and so on. Even worse than this is the use of asterisks in tables, with a footnote such as '[*] < 0.05', or '[**] < 0.01'. The authors should provide the actual *p*-value. Apart from anything else, it's useful to know how far from 0.05 it is. Note though, that some computer programs only give the *p*-value to three decimal places. So if a *p*-value = 0.0006, some programs will show this as $p = 0.000$, and authors can then only report this as '*p*-value <0.001.

MAKING THE WRONG DECISION – TYPES OF ERROR

We need to say a just few words about possible types of error in hypothesis testing because there is a connection to the power of a test (discussed in Chapter 8). It's worth bearing in mind that when researchers report the decision to reject or not reject the null hypothesis on the basis of some *sample* evidence, there is always the possibility that they might, unwittingly, have made the *wrong* decision, either because the sample is not representative enough of the population, or is not big enough to detect an effect. There are two scenarios: Type I errors and Type II errors.

Type I Errors

First, they may conclude from the sample data that the evidence against the null hypothesis is strong enough (*p*-value less than 0.05) for it to be rejected as false when it is in fact true. Statisticians refer to this mistake as a *Type I error*, although the term 'false positive' may be more familiar to you.

There are three common reasons for researchers to get a false positive result from a study. First, they may choose a biased sample which is not representative of the study population. Second, they may take too small a sample, so that a false positive result is obtained by chance. Both these sources of error can be eliminated by careful attention to sampling (see Chapter 8). Third, and harder to spot or deal with, is the possibility of false positive results arising from *multiple testing*.

You will remember that the *p*-value is the probability of a result occurring by chance and conventionally we accept $p < 0.05$ implying significance. What this means is that there is only a 5% likelihood of a result being due to chance, that is 1 in 20. But many studies report the results of more than 20 significance tests! Bear in mind, then, that if authors accept a significance level of $p < 0.05$ and conduct 20 tests, one of them at least may be 'positive' simply by chance.

Researchers can combine these errors by undertaking lots of subgroup analysis on their data. Subgroups are (by definition) smaller than the original sample, so chance may produce positive results, and the additional analyses involve more tests so multiple testing becomes a problem.

Type II Errors

The second possibility is that investigators may decide that the evidence against the null hypothesis is *not* strong enough for it to be rejected as being untrue (*p*-value not less than 0.05), when in fact it *is* untrue and the null hypothesis should have been rejected. Again the vagaries of samples might cause this to occur from time to time. Statisticians know this sort of mistake as a *Type II error*, or 'false negative'.

False negative results mainly occur as the result of studies which are too small. For example, suppose we want to know if women are on average shorter than men. If we take a sample of five women and five men we might easily find five tall women and five short men by chance, and conclude (wrongly) that women are not shorter than men. If we take a sample of 500 in each group we are much less likely to make this mistake (although we might still do so if the sample is biased).

This is where the power of a study comes in. The probability of committing a Type II error, of getting a false negative, is designated β. The *power* of a test is its ability to detect a true effect if such an effect exists; that is, to *avoid* not rejecting the null hypothesis when it is not true. Thus the power of a study equals $(1 - \beta)$ and it is intimately connected with the size of a study – larger studies have more power. Look again at Chapter 8 if you need to review the concept of power. If authors are presenting the results of hypothesis tests, they must provide evidence that a power calculation to determine the minimum sample size needed to detect the condition has been performed.

Even if the researchers intend to analyse their results using confidence intervals without performing any tests, the sample size calculation still needs to be done. The problem of too small a sample manifests itself in confidence intervals by producing wide intervals with little precision. These may fail to pick up a significant result (i.e. give a false negative).

HYPOTHESIS TESTS AND CONFIDENCE INTERVALS COMPARED

Confidence intervals and hypothesis tests perform a similar function. For example, in the bone mineral density (BMD) study referred to above (and also considered in Figure 19.1 in the context of confidence intervals), the research question was, 'Is the bone mineral density the same in depressed and non-depressed women?' We know that this question can be answered in two ways, either by calculating a confidence interval for the *difference* in mean bone mineral densities and seeing if it contains 0, or by testing the null hypothesis that the difference in mean bone mineral densities is equal to zero, and seeing if the *p*-value is less than 0.05. In fact, if the 95% confidence interval includes 0, the *p*-value will equal 0.05 or more; if the confidence interval doesn't contain 0, the *p*-value will be less than 0.05.

If authors provide both *p*-values and confidence intervals for a test, you should find they that they display this sort of agreement. Note, however, as we saw in Chapter 20, that if the paper deals with the testing of *ratios*, then the *p*-value will be less than 0.05 if the 95% confidence does *not* include 1 (and vice versa). There is an example of this later in the chapter. Confidence intervals are preferred because they also provide a *range of plausible values* for the size of any difference, whereas the hypothesis test only indicates whether any difference is statistically significant, but without any indication of what that difference might be.

Take, for example, the result for the difference in mean bone mineral densities at the lumbar spine, shown in the first row of Figure 21.1 (this is the same study first encountered in Figure 19.1). The *p*-value is 0.02, which is quite strong enough for us to reject the null hypothesis of equal mean BMDs in the two populations. But that's all it tells us. However, the confidence interval of (0.02 to 0.14) g/cm^2

BONE MINERAL DENSITY IN WOMEN WITH DEPRESSION

DAVID MICHELSON, M.D., CONSTANTINE STRATAKIS, M.D., PHD., LAUREN HILL, B.S., JAMES REYNOLDS, M.D., ELISE GALLIVEN, B.S., GEORGE CHROUSOS, M.D., AND PHILIP GOLD M.D.

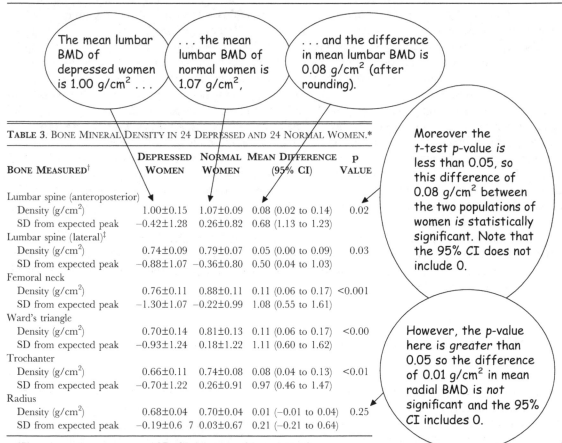

The mean lumbar BMD of depressed women is 1.00 g/cm^2 . . .

. . . the mean lumbar BMD of normal women is 1.07 g/cm^2,

. . . and the difference in mean lumbar BMD is 0.08 g/cm^2 (after rounding).

Moreover the t-test p-value *is* less than 0.05, so this difference of 0.08 g/cm^2 between the two populations of women *is* statistically significant. Note that the 95% CI does not include 0.

However, the p-value here is *greater* than 0.05 so the difference of 0.01 g/cm^2 in mean radial BMD is *not* significant and the 95% CI includes 0.

TABLE 3. BONE MINERAL DENSITY IN 24 DEPRESSED AND 24 NORMAL WOMEN.*

BONE MEASURED[†]	DEPRESSED WOMEN	NORMAL WOMEN	MEAN DIFFERENCE (95% CI)	p VALUE
Lumbar spine (anteroposterior)				
Density (g/cm^2)	1.00±0.15	1.07±0.09	0.08 (0.02 to 0.14)	0.02
SD from expected peak	−0.42±1.28	0.26±0.82	0.68 (1.13 to 1.23)	
Lumbar spine (lateral)[‡]				
Density (g/cm^2)	0.74±0.09	0.79±0.07	0.05 (0.00 to 0.09)	0.03
SD from expected peak	−0.88±1.07	−0.36±0.80	0.50 (0.04 to 1.03)	
Femoral neck				
Density (g/cm^2)	0.76±0.11	0.88±0.11	0.11 (0.06 to 0.17)	<0.001
SD from expected peak	−1.30±1.07	−0.22±0.99	1.08 (0.55 to 1.61)	
Ward's triangle				
Density (g/cm^2)	0.70±0.14	0.81±0.13	0.11 (0.06 to 0.17)	<0.00
SD from expected peak	−0.93±1.24	0.18±1.22	1.11 (0.60 to 1.62)	
Trochanter				
Density (g/cm^2)	0.66±0.11	0.74±0.08	0.08 (0.04 to 0.13)	<0.01
SD from expected peak	−0.70±1.22	0.26±0.91	0.97 (0.46 to 1.47)	
Radius				
Density (g/cm^2)	0.68±0.04	0.70±0.04	0.01 (−0.01 to 0.04)	0.25
SD from expected peak	−0.19±0.6 7	0.03±0.67	0.21 (−0.21 to 0.64)	

*Plus-minus values are means ±SD. CI denotes confidence interval.

[†]Values for "SD from expected peak" are the numbers of standard deviations from the expected peak density derived from a population-based study of normal white women.[3]

[‡]This measurement was made in 23 depressed women and 23 normal women.

FIGURE 21.1   Differences in mean bone mineral density in depressed and normal women, and corresponding *p*-values

tells us not only that the mean BMDs are different, because the confidence interval does not include 0, but also that a plausible value for this difference most probably lies between 0.02 and 0.14 g/cm^2.

A further important reason for preferring to see authors using the confidence interval approach to that of hypothesis testing is that the plausible range of value provided is in clinically meaningful units, which of course makes interpretation much easier. Far better for you to know that 'the difference in mean lumbar bone mineral density is most probably between 0.02 and 0.14 g/cm^2', than just to be told that '$p = 0.034$'.

TYPES OF TEST

Matched versus Independent Groups

Like much else we have discussed so far, the choice by researchers of an appropriate statistical test when two groups are involved is governed not only by the type of data in question and the shape of the distributions. In addition, for hypothesis testing we also need to know whether the groups involved are *independent* or *matched* (the word 'paired' is also used as a synonym for matched). For groups to be independent, the selection of the subjects for one group must not be influenced by or related to the selection of subjects for the other group. However, there are occasions when groups might be matched, for example, in some case–control studies (see Chapter 5).

This matching can be on a person-to-person basis, or in proportinial terms (for example, the same proportion of males to females in each group, the same proportion of those aged over 60, and so on). So, when the results of any test on two groups appears in a paper, you should be able to tell whether or not the groups were matched. If matched, what is the nature of the matching – individual-to-individual or by proportion? If the latter, then the groups are not considered to be matched for the purpose of hypothesis testing. If the groups are supposedly independent you will want evidence that this is true. In either case, you will also want to know exactly how many were in each group. There are numerous different statistical tests in common use in the clinical literature. However, we will briefly describe the three tests which appear most often in non-specialist clinical papers: the chi-squared test, the Mann-Whitney test, and the *t*-test.

The Chi-squared (χ^2) Test

Suppose you take a sample of male nurses and female nurses working in a large hospital, and record whether or not they smoke. You want to answer the question, 'Is there a relationship between sex and smoking status or are these two variables independent?' In other words, are you more (or less) likely to smoke if you are female (say) than if you are male, or doesn't gender make any difference? Your null hypothesis is that the variables are independent – gender and smoking are not related. You can express this problem as a 2×2 *contingency* table (a table containing the observed frequencies). If the null hypothesis is true, if the variables *are* independent, then the proportion of males in each category (smoking, and non-smoking), should be approximately the same as the proportion of females in each category. However, since we are dealing with sample data, the sample proportions are unlikely to be *exactly* the same even if the null hypothesis is true. We can use the *chi-squared test* to determine whether any observed differences in the proportions exceed what we might expect by chance. One condition of the test is that the observations on the two (or more) groups, in this case male nurses and female nurses, *must be independent*. The above example had two categories (smokers and non-smokers, and two groups, males and females), and would be referred to as a 2×2 test, but chi-squared can be used with more than two groups and/or categories, as you will see below.

The test can be used with data of any type, but in practice it is most often applied to nominal or ordinal data, provided that the number of categories is not too large; chi-squared is seldom used with more than four or five categories. In fact, the number of categories is limited by the size of the sample. The reasons behind this are a bit technical, but as a rough guide with two groups and three categories you would need a minimum total sample of 50 or upwards (authors should, of course, give evidence of a power calculation, see Chapter 8). Sample size considerations and the need for the groups to be independent are something to be aware of when you read papers containing chi-squared results.

As an example, the next study was an investigation of the merits of three different prescribing strategies for sore throat. Group 1 were given a prescription for antibiotics for 10 days. Group 2 were not given a prescription. Group 3 were given a prescription for antibiotics if symptoms were not starting to settle down after 3 days. Apart from the clinical aspects of the study, patients were also given a questionnaire and asked to score, 'very', 'moderately', 'slightly', or 'not at all', to a number of questions.

The authors wanted to know, for each question asked, whether the combined percentage of patients answering 'very' or 'moderately' compared with the combined percentage answering 'slightly' or 'not at all', was the same (the null hypothesis) in Groups 1, 2 and 3. In other words, is satisfaction with the consultation related to group (i.e. to prescribing strategy) or not? The differences between the percentages were tested using the chi-squared test and the results are shown in Figure 21.2.

Figure 21.2 shows that the sample percentages answering 'very' or 'moderately' to the question, 'Were you satisfied with your consultation?' are 96% in Group 1, 90% in Group 2, and 93% in Group 3. The null hypothesis is that in the population these percentages are the same, and although the percentages do appear very similar, we need the chi-squared test to tell us formally whether the observed differences are statistically significant. The p-value for the chi-squared test is given in the table as 0.09, which is not less than 0.05 (as expected) so does not offer sufficiently strong evidence to enable us to reject the null hypothesis. There appears to be a similar degree of satisfaction with the consultation in all three groups.

Note that the p-value of 0.09 implies that we can be 91% certain (1.00 minus 0.09 = 0.91, or 91%) that there is a difference between the percentages in each group who are satisfied with their consultation. However, since we have set a benchmark p-value of 0.05 (which 0.09 exceeds) we *cannot* conclude that these differences are statistically significant. They are reasonably likely to be due to chance alone.

If we consider the responses of the three groups to the question, 'Are antibiotics effective?' shown on the fourth row of the table, we see a p-value of 0.001. This tells us that there *is* a relationship between belief in the effectiveness of antibiotics and prescribing strategy (i.e. we can reject the null hypothesis). Put another way, this means that the proportions in each category (each prescribing group) are not the same, but the test does not tell us what the actual group population percents or proportions might be. The best estimates are the sample percentages. For example, 87% of those given antibiotics (Group 1), believed they were effective, and this would be the best-guess for the percentage in this group in the population with this belief. More useful (as we now know) would have been confidence intervals for these percentages which would then offer us a range of plausible values for the true percentage. Unfortunately the authors do not provide these.

The Chi-squared Test with Odds Ratios, Risk Ratios, etc.

A second use you will see for the chi-squared test is as a measure of the statistical significance of odds and risk ratios and the like, in the study of potential risk factors for various conditions. If we use the p-value to test hypotheses related to a ratio, for example, an odds ratio, then as you saw above, a p-value of less than 0.05 will correspond to a confidence interval for the ratio that does not include 1.

Open randomised trial of prescribing strategies in managing sore throat

P Little, I Williamson, G Warner, C Gould, M Gantley, A L Kinmonth

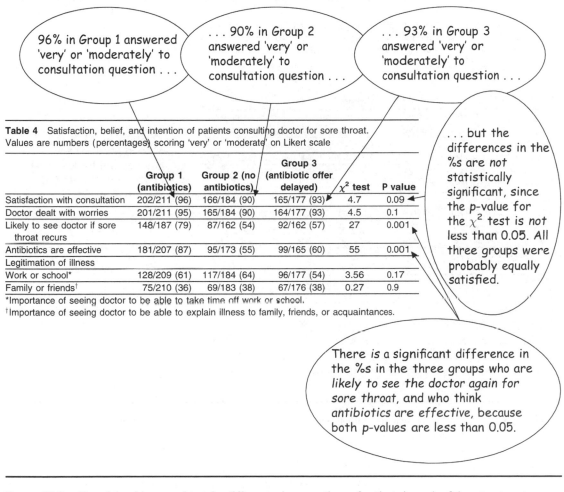

96% in Group 1 answered 'very' or 'moderately' to consultation question . . .

. . . 90% in Group 2 answered 'very' or 'moderately' to consultation question . . .

. . . 93% in Group 3 answered 'very' or 'moderately' to consultation question . . .

Table 4 Satisfaction, belief, and intention of patients consulting doctor for sore throat. Values are numbers (percentages) scoring 'very' or 'moderate' on Likert scale

	Group 1 (antibiotics)	Group 2 (no antibiotics)	Group 3 (antibiotic offer delayed)	χ^2 test	P value
Satisfaction with consultation	202/211 (96)	166/184 (90)	165/177 (93)	4.7	0.09
Doctor dealt with worries	201/211 (95)	165/184 (90)	164/177 (93)	4.5	0.1
Likely to see doctor if sore throat recurs	148/187 (79)	87/162 (54)	92/162 (57)	27	0.001
Antibiotics are effective	181/207 (87)	95/173 (55)	99/165 (60)	55	0.001
Legitimation of illness					
Work or school*	128/209 (61)	117/184 (64)	96/177 (54)	3.56	0.17
Family or friends†	75/210 (36)	69/183 (38)	67/176 (38)	0.27	0.9

*Importance of seeing doctor to be able to take time off work or school.
†Importance of seeing doctor to be able to explain illness to family, friends, or acquaintances.

. . . but the differences in the %s are not statistically significant, since the p-value for the χ^2 test is not less than 0.05. All three groups were probably equally satisfied.

There *is* a significant difference in the %s in the three groups who are likely to see the doctor again for sore throat, and who think antibiotics are effective, because both p-values are less than 0.05.

FIGURE 21.2   Use of the chi-squared test for differences in proportions of patients in each of three treatment groups answering 'very' or 'moderately' to a number of questions in a sore throat study

As an example, Figure 21.3 is taken from a study into the use of brief integrin β_3 for long-term protection against myocardial ischaemic events (the same study as in Figure 11.3). Subjects were randomized into three groups. The first group received an abciximab* bolus followed by an abciximab infusion for 12 hours; the second group an abciximab bolus followed by a placebo infusion; the third group a placebo bolus plus a placebo infusion.

—————————

*Abciximab is an antibody fragment which prevents platelet aggregation.

Long-term Protection from Myocardial Ischemic Events in a Randomized Trial of Brief Integrin β_3 Blockade with Percutaneous Coronary Intervention

Eric J. Topol, MD; James J. Ferguson, MD; Harlan F. Weisman, MD; James E. Tcheng, MD; Stephen G. Ellis, MD; Neal S. Kleiman, MD; Russell J. Ivanhoe, MD; Ann L. Wang; David P. Miller, MS; Keaven M. Anderson, PhD; Robert M. Califf, MD; for the EPIC Investigator Group

Table 3.—Clinical Outcomes: Death/Myocardial Infarction/Any Coronary Revascularization*

End point	Placebo (n=696)	Bolus (n=698)	Bolus + infusion (n=708)	P Value	Odds Ratio (95% Confidence Interval)
Composite					
1 year	266 (38.6)	251 (36.3)	216 (30.8)	.002	0.75 (0.63–0.90)
2 years	290 (42.3)	290 (42.4)	253 (36.3)	.009	0.80 (0.68–0.95)
3 years	319 (47.2)	321 (47.4)	284 (41.1)	.009	0.81 (0.69–0.95)
Death					
1 year	31 (4.5)	29 (4.2)	30 (4.2)	.841	0.95 (0.58–1.57)
2 years	46 (6.6)	40 (5.8)	37 (5.2)	.277	0.79 (0.51–1.22)
3 years	59 (8.6)	54 (8.0)	47 (6.8)	.202	0.78 (0.53–1.14)
Myocardial infarction					
1 year	77 (11.2)	62 (9.0)	55 (7.9)	.032	0.69 (0.49–0.97)
2 years	84 (12.4)	73 (10.8)	64 (9.3)	.057	0.73 (0.53–1.01)
3 years	91 (13.6)	81 (12.2)	72 (10.7)	.075	0.76 (0.56–1.03)
Revascularization					
1 year	221 (32.6)	207 (30.4)	178 (25.6)	.004	0.75 (0.62–0.91)
2 years	242 (36.0)	237 (35.3)	207 (30.2)	.013	0.79 (0.66–0.95)
3 years	265 (40.1)	256 (38.6)	234 (34.8)	.021	0.81 (0.68–0.97)

With a ratio (such as the odds ratio) the p-value will be less than 0.05 when the 95% CI does not include 1, . . .

. . . and vice versa.

*P value and odds ratio represent the comparison of bolus + infusion vs placebo. All values are No. (%) except where otherwise indicated.

FIGURE 21.3 Odds ratios for various clinical outcomes in a comparison of integrin β_3 with placebo for long-term protection from myocardial events

End-points of interest included: (1) a composite of death, myocardial infarction or revascularisation; (2) death; (3) myocardial infarction; and (4) revascularisation. These were examined at one, two and three years. Figure 21.3 sets out the odds ratios for the comparison of bolus plus infusion versus placebo, along with 95% confidence intervals and *p*-values. Notice that the *p*-values are less than 0.05 when the 95% confidence intervals for the odds ratios do not include 1.

The Chi-squared Test for Trend

A third use for the chi-squared test is to test for trends in the proportions or percentages across categories when the categories are ordered. Note that establishing a linear trend across categories implies a relationship between the two variables in question, but the chi-squared test for trend is more powerful than the 'ordinary' chi-squared test described above and authors should use it whenever categories can be

Relation of exposure to airway irritants in infancy to prevalence of bronchial hyper-responsiveness in schoolchildren

Vidar Søyseth, Johny Kongerud, Dagfinn Haarr, Ole Strand, Roald Bolle, Jacob Boe

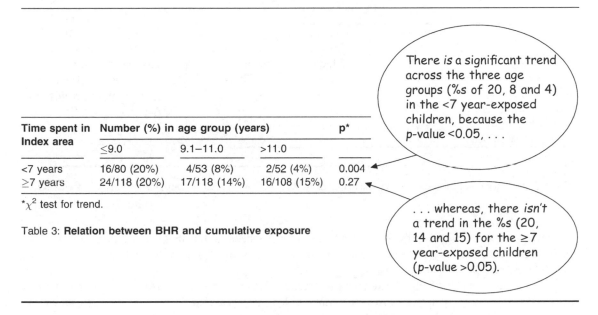

Time spent in Index area	Number (%) in age group (years)			p*
	≤9.0	9.1–11.0	>11.0	
<7 years	16/80 (20%)	4/53 (8%)	2/52 (4%)	0.004
≥7 years	24/118 (20%)	17/118 (14%)	16/108 (15%)	0.27

*χ^2 test for trend.

Table 3: **Relation between BHR and cumulative exposure**

> There *is* a significant trend across the three age groups (%s of 20, 8 and 4) in the <7 year-exposed children, because the *p*-value <0.05, . . .

> . . . whereas, there *isn't* a trend in the %s (20, 14 and 15) for the ≥7 year-exposed children (*p*-value >0.05).

FIGURE 21.4 An example of the use of the chi-squared test for trend across three age-groups among two groups of children

ordered. For example, the categories might be the age-groups (0–19, 20–29, etc.), whereas the two groups might be depressed and not depressed patients. The chi-squared test for trend could then be used to discover whether or not there was a *systematic* trend in the proportion depressed as age-group increased.

Figure 21.4 shows the results of a chi-squared test to determine whether there was a trend in the percentages of children exposed to air pollution in two groups across three age-groups. One group had been exposed for less than seven years, the other for seven years or more. The chi-squared test is a very versatile procedure and has several other important applications, for example, in meta-analysis (see Chapter 26) and in logistic regression (see Chapter 25).

The Mann-Whitney Test

The Mann-Whitney test (sometimes the Mann-Whitney U test), is commonly used to decide whether the medians of two *independent* groups are the same or not. It is a popular alternative to the *t*-test (see next section) if the requirements of the *t*-test (metric data, Normally distributed) cannot be met. It is most often used therefore with either ordinal data or skewed metric data. The method combines the values in the two groups and then ranks them (while preserving the group identity of each ranked value). The sum of the ranks in each group is calculated and if the null hypothesis of equal medians is true, then we would expect these two rank sums to be similar. The Mann-Whitney test tells us whether the observed difference

Depressive symptoms in long-term care residents in Taiwan

Li-Chan Lin, Tyng-Guey Wang, Miao-Yen Chen, Shiao-Chi Wu and Portwood MJ

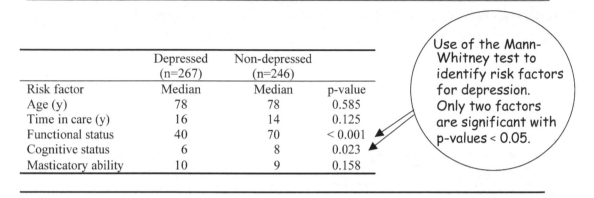

Risk factor	Depressed (n=267) Median	Non-depressed (n=246) Median	p-value
Age (y)	78	78	0.585
Time in care (y)	16	14	0.125
Functional status	40	70	< 0.001
Cognitive status	6	8	0.023
Masticatory ability	10	9	0.158

FIGURE 21.5   Results of a Mann-Whitney test to identify risk factors for depressive symptoms in elderly residents in care

in the two rank sums is greater than we might expect by chance, and thus that the two medicans may not be the same. Authors may sometimes quote a value for the Mann-Whitney 'U statistic', but this is of little interest compared to the corresponding *p*-value.

As an example of the Mann-Whitney test in practice Figure 21.5 is taken from a study into the risk factors for depressive symptoms in older people in long-term care in Taiwan. The figure shows the median values among depressed and a non-depressed groups for five potential risk factors, along with a *p*-value from a Mann-Whitney *test of equal medians*. Although the first two factors, age and length of time in care, are metric variables and, distributional requirements permitting, could have been tested using a 2-sample *t*-test (see next section), the other three factors are ordinal. In any case, the authors have used the Mann-Whitney test with all five factors. As you can see, only two factors, Functional status and Cognitive status, are statistically significant risk factors for depressive symptoms, with *p*-values of <0.001 and 0.023 respectively.

The *t*-test

The *t*-test is most often used with metric data to test for a difference in means between two groups. If the groups are matched or paired, the matched-pairs *t*-test is used; if independent, the two-sample *t*-test is used. If the two-sample *t*-test is used, the data in both groups must be metric and Normally distributed. In addition, the standard deviations of each group should be similar – as a rule-of-thumb, one standard deviation should be no more than twice the other. Authors seldom provide evidence that they have examined the shape of their distributions before using the 2-sample *t*-test, although with large samples this precaution becomes less crucial.

Transforming Data

If the data are not Normal, the authors may report that they *transformed* it to achieve approximate Normality, prior to applying the test. This transformation will often also improve the similarity of the standard deviations. The most common transformation is the $\log_{10}$ transformation, not only because it is successful more often than other possible transformations, but also because the back-transformation (by anti-logging) at the end of the analysis can be meaningfully interpreted. It is important to understand that when authors are examining the difference between two means and have log-transformed the data, the back-transformation produces a *ratio*.

For example, imagine we are using the 2-sample *t*-test to examine the difference in mean age of male and female trainee nurses in a new intake, and we have had to log transform the data to make it more Normal. Suppose the log results give us a difference in log means (males – females), of 0.078 with a 95% log confidence interval of (0.0715 to 0.0846). When we back-transform by anti-logging we get a difference in means of 1.197 with a 95% confidence interval of (1.179 to 1.215). The correct interpretation of this result is that the mean age of the male nurses is 19.7% *greater* than the mean age of the female nurses, with a 95% confidence interval for the *ratio* of mean ages, of from 17.9% greater to 21.5% greater.

If the matched-pairs *t*-test is used, then there is no requirement for each either group to have Normally distributed data, but the *differences* between the two sets of data must be Normally distributed. For example, in testing the difference between the mean bone mineral densities (Figure 21.1), the two groups of normal and depressed women were matched so authors used the matched-pairs *t*-test. The *p*-values given in Figure 21.1 are therefore for these six matched-pairs *t*-tests.

As an example of the 2-sample *t*-test, Figure 21.6 is from a randomized trial comparing laparoscopy-assisted colectomy versus open colectomy for the treatment of non-metastatic colon cancer. The authors used the 2-sample *t*-test to compare the differences in means between the two groups for a number of outcomes. Since these outcomes are metric and the groups independent, the 2-sample *t*-test is appropriate. The authors do not comment on the shape of any of the distributions in their paper but do provide information on the size of the standard deviations in the figure. Notice that there is a statistically significant difference for all outcomes shown (all *p*-values <0.05).

Laparoscopy-assisted colectomy versus open colectomy for treatment of non-metastatic colon cancer: a randomised trial

Antonio M Lacy, Juan C Garcia-Valdecasas, Salvadora Delgado, Antoni Castells, Pilar Taura, Joseph M Pique, Joseph Visa

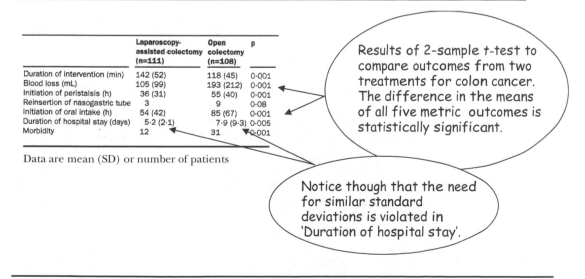

	Laparoscopy-assisted colectomy (n=111)	Open colectomy (n=108)	p
Duration of intervention (min)	142 (52)	118 (45)	0·001
Blood loss (mL)	105 (99)	193 (212)	0·001
Initiation of peristalsis (h)	36 (31)	55 (40)	0·001
Reinsertion of nasogastric tube	3	9	0·08
Initiation of oral intake (h)	54 (42)	85 (67)	0·001
Duration of hospital stay (days)	5·2 (2·1)	7·9 (9·3)	0·005
Morbidity	12	31	0·001

Data are mean (SD) or number of patients

Results of 2-sample *t*-test to compare outcomes from two treatments for colon cancer. The difference in the means of all five metric outcomes is statistically significant.

Notice though that the need for similar standard deviations is violated in 'Duration of hospital stay'.

FIGURE 21.6   Results of two-sample *t*-test to compare outcomes from two treatment for colon cancer. Note that re-insertion of nasogastric tube and morbidity were compare using a chi-squared test

TABLE 21.1   A few of the more common statistical tests

The two-sample *t*-test	Most often used to test for difference in *means* of two *independent* groups. Both sets of data must be metric and Normally distributed, and have similar standard deviations (as a rule of thumb one not more than twice the other).
The matched-pairs *t-test*	Most often used to test for difference in *means* of two *matched* groups. Data must be metric and differences between group scores Normally distributed.
The 1-way analysis of variance (Anova) test	Most often used to test for differences in the means of three or more groups. Data must be metric and Normally distributed in each group and all standard deviations must be similar.
The Mann-Whitney test	Most often used to test for difference in *medians* of two *independent* groups. Data can be either ordinal or metric (any shape distributions but must be similar in each group).
The Wilcoxon test	Most often used to test for difference in *medians* of two *matched* groups. Data can be either ordinal or metric (any shape distribution but differences in scores must be distributed approximately symmetrically).
The chi-squared test	Most often used to measure whether two variables are *independent* or not; does this by comparing differences in proportions across categories. Data must be categorical (or categorised metric) and groups independent. When sample size is small, the chi-squared test may not be appropriate. In a two-group, two-category case, Fisher's test may be used instead. The same data conditions apply.
The chi-squared test for trend	Most often used to determine whether there is a systematic *trend* in proportions across categories. Data must be categorical (or categorised metric).
The McNemar test	Most often used to measure the difference in *proportions* (or percentages) of two *matched* groups across two categories. Data can be nominal or ordinal.
The Kruskal-Wallis test	Most often used to test whether the *medians* of three or more independent groups are the same. Data can be ordinal or metric (any shape distributions but must be similar in each group).

Finally . . .

There are dozens, perhaps hundreds, of statistical tests which at some time may appear in clinical journals. Obviously we have discussed only a few of the most commonly used. Specialist areas of clinical research will use more specialist tests. The more common tests in the generalist journals are described very briefly in Table 21.1, along with the required data type and distributional (shape) requirements.

Note that the first two tests in Table 21.1 (the 2-sample and matched-pairs *t*-tests), are *parametric* tests. That is, they have precise distributional requirements – data needs to be Normally distributed. The remaining tests in the table are *non-parametric* – they have no such precise distributional requirements.

In short, the authors should tell you which tests they have used (and why) to get the results they present. With the help of Table 21.1 you should be able to judge whether the chosen test is appropriate. For example, in the following study the authors were describing a randomized controlled trial to compare the clinical efficacy of midwife-managed care (midwife only) for pregnant women, with shared care (midwives plus doctors). Their methods section contained a brief summary of the statistical methods employed (Figure 21.7).

Randomised, controlled trial of efficacy of midwife-managed care

Deborah Turnbull, Ann Holmes, Noreen Shields, Helen Cheyne, Sara Twaddle, W Harper Gilmour, Mary McGinley, Margaret Reid, Irene Johnstone, Ian Geer, Gillian McIlwaine, C Burnett Lunan

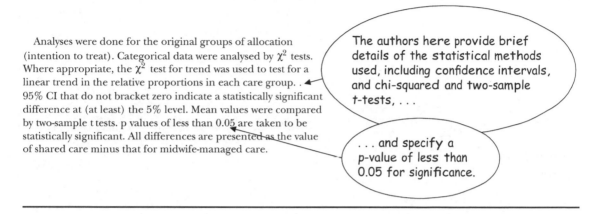

Analyses were done for the original groups of allocation (intention to treat). Categorical data were analysed by χ^2 tests. Where appropriate, the χ^2 test for trend was used to test for a linear trend in the relative proportions in each care group. . 95% CI that do not bracket zero indicate a statistically significant difference at (at least) the 5% level. Mean values were compared by two-sample t tests. p values of less than 0.05 are taken to be statistically significant. All differences are presented as the value of shared care minus that for midwife-managed care.

The authors here provide brief details of the statistical methods used, including confidence intervals, and chi-squared and two-sample t-tests, . . .

. . . and specify a p-value of less than 0.05 for significance.

FIGURE 21.7   Description by authors of types of statistical tests used in a midwife-managed care study

VII

Analysing the Data:
Multivariable Methods

22

Measuring Association

The various types of statistical analysis we have considered so far have involved only a *single* variable, usually measured in two or more groups, for example, bone mineral density in normal and depressed women, the degree of stump pain in treatment and placebo groups, childhood mortality by social grouping, and so on. On many occasions, however, researchers want to measure the degree of 'connection' between two or more variables; for example, between systolic blood pressure *and* body mass index, or between coronary heart disease *and* exercise. One possible approach is for them to measure what is called the *association* between the two variables. By association we mean the way that two variables appear to move together. This is what we are going to look at in this chapter.

Less frequently authors may want to measure how well the scores on two variables *agree*, for example, blood pressure measurements on the same patients by two different practice nurses, or answers given by patients to a questionnaire today and three months ago. We discuss ways of measuring agreement in Chapter 23.

Papers can be found in which association is sometimes employed as a proxy for agreement. However, there is a fundamental difference between the two measures, as we shall see. To illustrate the difference, suppose a trainee paramedic assesses the Glasgow Coma Scale score of 10 patients. His supervisor simultaneously scores the same patients. Their scores are:

Patient	1	2	3	4	5	6	7	8	9	10
Trainee	5	9	3	7	8	5	4	9	7	5
Supervisor	4	8	2	5	8	4	2	8	6	5

We can see that when the supervisor scores high, the trainee also tends to score high. When the supervisor scores low, the trainee tends to score low. The two sets of scores seem to be positively associated. *Positively* associated, because when the trainee gives a high score, the supervisor also tends to give a high score (and similarly low scores tend to be associated with low scores).

The opposite situation (high scores with low scores, and vice versa) is called *negative association* (we'll come to an example of this shortly). The *strength* of any association between sets of scores will vary from weak or non-existent, through moderate, to strong, and may be positive or negative. So how can we measure association?

HOW CAN WE MEASURE ASSOCIATION?

The Scatter Diagram

One simple (but non-quantitative) method authors sometimes use for assessing the strength and direction of an association is to plot a *scatter diagram* (or scattergram) of the data. If we do this for the Glasgow Coma Scale scores, we get the graph shown in Figure 22.1.

Understanding Clinical Papers Second Edition David Bowers, Allan House, David Owens
© 2006 John Wiley & Sons, Ltd

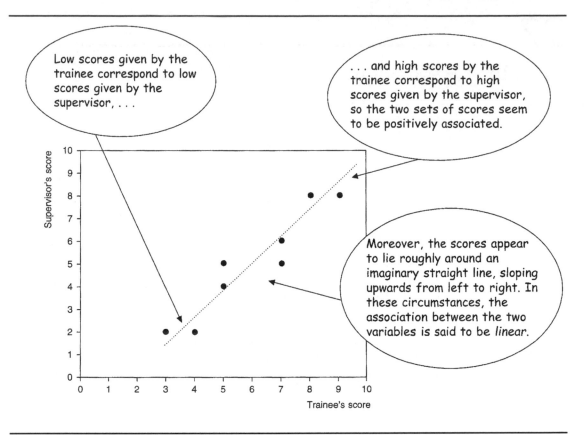

FIGURE 22.1 Scattergram of hypothetical GCS scores given to 10 patients by supervisor and trainee paramedic

A real example is shown below from a study into hospital league tables. The scatter diagram (Figure 22.2) shows the percentage mortality from aortic aneurysm in each of 18 hospitals, plotted against the annual number of episodes of this condition treated by each hospital. It is apparent that the two variables are negatively associated. In general, hospitals that dealt with low numbers of episodes had high mortality rates, hospitals with high numbers of episodes had low mortality rates (one possible explanation for this is that the more experience the hospital had in dealing with the condition, the lower the mortality rate, and vice versa).

The *strength* of any association depends on how close the points are to lying on an imaginary straight line. The closer they are, the stronger the association. If all the points fell *exactly* on the line, the association would be described as *perfect*. Of course, with sample data this never happens. With the aortic aneurysm data (if we leave out the point lying on the horizontal axis, as being a possible outlier), then we can imagine a straight line drawn through the scatter, which would slope down from left to right, but clearly not all of the points can fall on this line. Note that when the points do lie approximately around a straight line, the association between the two variables is said to be *linear* (more on linear relationships in Chapter 24).

Mortality league tables: do they inform or mislead?

Martin McKee, Duncan Hunter

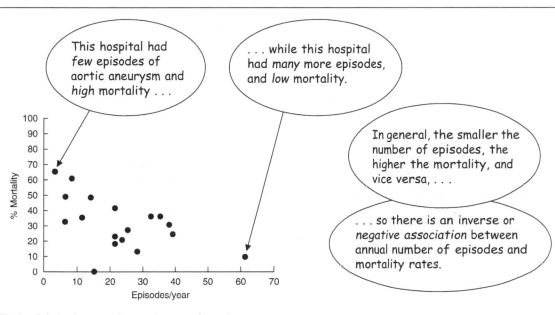

Fig 3   Relation between volume and outcome for aortic aneurysm

FIGURE 22.2   Scattergram of percentage mortality from aortic aneurysm in 16 hospitals against number of episodes dealt with per year

This idea may be clearer in Figure 22.3, taken from a study which compared, for a large number of patients, the patients' own *estimation* of their body mass index (BMI) with an accurate *measurement* taken in a clinic. The two sets of measurements seem to be positively associated, with low estimated body mass indexes associated with low measured body mass indexes, and vice versa. The 'best' straight line drawn through the points shows that the majority of them lie on or close to the line, indicating a linear association. Thus we would judge the association to be strong (and positive).

However, eyeballing a scatter diagram to judge the strength of an association, although often insightful, suffers severe limitations (for example if we want to judge the *relative* strengths of two associations). For this reason, researchers usually turn to a quantitative measure.

THE CORRELATION COEFFICIENT

The correlation coefficient is the most widely used quantitative measure of association. It is a single numeric measure of the strength of the *linear* association between two variables. There may well be a strong association between two variables which is *not* linear (for example, it might be exponential), but a correlation coefficient of the type discussed here may not detect this as a strong association (or any association at all). Authors most often use either *Pearson's* correlation coefficient (denoted *r*) or

GP documentation of obesity: what does it achieve?

PAUL LITTLE

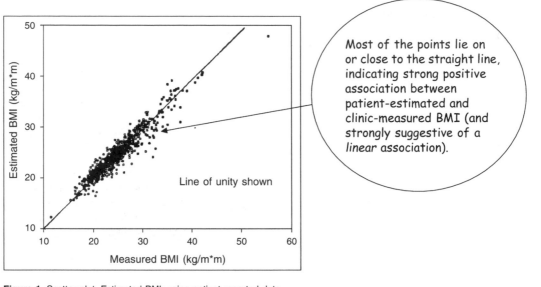

Figure 1. Scatter plot. Estimated BMI: using patient reported data.
Measured BMI: using staiometer and scales.

FIGURE 22.3   Scattergram of estimated against measured body mass index

Spearman's correlation coefficient (denoted r_S), both of which are similarly interpreted. Both r and r_S can vary between -1 (indicating perfect negative association) and $+1$ (indicating perfect positive association). The further away from 0 the coefficient is (in either direction), the stronger the association.

The correlation coefficients r and r_S, calculated from sample data, are of course only *estimates* of the true (population) correlation coefficients. To measure the statistical significance of the true (population) correlation coefficient (statistical inference again), authors can either present confidence intervals or *p*-values, with the usual rules for significance applying; i.e. confidence intervals not including zero or *p*-values less than 0.05 (see Chapters 19 and 21).

Choice of the most appropriate correlation coefficient is governed by the same considerations of data type and distributional shape as the measures considered in preceding units, so you need to be able to tell what type of data the authors are using and what shape the two distributions concerned have. The rule which authors should follow is:

to calculate Pearson's r, and obtain a confidence interval both sets of data should be metric and (approximately) Normally distributed. Failing this, or with either variable ordinal, Spearman's rank-based coefficient r_S should be used.

The authors in the following case–control study were comparing the reliability of medical records with maternally reported birth characteristics. The subjects in the study were mothers whose children had received a diagnosis of leukaemia at age 18 months. Figure 22.4 shows Pearson correlation

Medical Record Validation of Maternally Reported Birth Characteristics and Pregnancy-related Events: A Report from the Children's Cancer Group

Janet E. Olson,[1] Xiao Ou Shu,[1] Julie A. Ross,[1] Thomas Pendergrass,[2] and Leslie L. Robison[1]

TABLE 3. Validity and reliability of gestational age within specific demographic subgroupings among participating members from a United States and Canadian cooperative clinical trials group and matched controls, 1983–1988

This should be 95%.

An r = 0.839 shows strong positive association between recall and record of gestational age, among all subjects, . . .

. . . confirmed by a 95% CI which does not include 0, so the true r is statistically significant.

Association between records and recall seems to weaken (r decreases from 0.896 to 0.852) as time since childbirth increases.

Association is positive and significant across all subgroups (none of the CIs includes 0).

	Correlation of gestational age	98% CI*	Kappa statistic[†]
All gestational ages	0.839	0.817–0.859	0.62
Case/control status			
Cases	0.849	0.813–0.878	0.63
Controls	0.835	0.805–0.861	0.61
Education			
<High school	0.694	0.553–0.797	0.51
High school	0.833	0.790–0.868	0.63
>High school	0.835	0.804–0.861	0.62
Household income			
<$22,000	0.791	0.734–0.837	0.59
$22,000–$34,999	0.882	0.849–0.908	0.62
≥$35,000	0.843	0.800–0.877	0.65
Unknown	0.745	0.641–0.823	0.60
Time (years) from delivery to interview			
<2	0.896	0.862–0.921	0.64
2–3.9	0.821	0.784–0.852	0.63
4–5.9	0.828	0.775–0.869	0.61
6–8	0.852	0.734–0.920	0.42
Maternal age (years)			
<25	0.822	0.773–0.861	0.64
25–29	0.889	0.862–0.912	0.63
30–34	0.760	0.694–0.813	0.57
≥35	0.888	0.824–0.930	0.64
Birth order			
First born	0.880	0.853–0.903	0.67
Second born	0.815	0.778–0.846	0.57
≥Third born	0.632	0.416–0.781	0.52
Maternal race			
White	0.846	0.822–0.866	0.64
Other	0.782	0.680–0.855	0.42

* CI, confidence interval.
[†] Three categories, <38, 38–41, ≥42 weeks.

FIGURE 22.4 Correlation of gestational age of child from medical records and as recalled by mother, according to a number of factors

coefficients for the association between the gestational age of the child concerned taken from clinical records and as recalled by the mother up to 4 years after childbirth (ignore the last column). Since gestational age is metric, Pearson's r is appropriate, provided that both sets of data are also Normally distributed (unfortunately there is no evidence that the authors have addressed this distributional issue).

In the next (cross-sectional) study (Figure 22.5), the authors were investigating the link between breast size and hormone levels, body constitution and oral contraceptive use. Although all the variables concerned (except for family history of breast cancer) are metric continuous, they have

Breast Size in Relation to Endogenous Hormone Levels, Body Constitution, and Oral Contraceptive Use in Healthy Nulligravid Women Aged 19–25 Years

Helena Jernström and Håkan Olsson

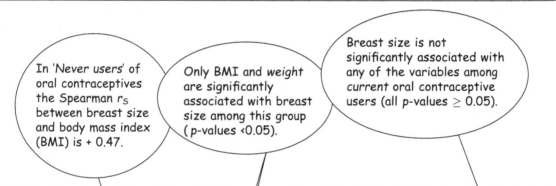

In 'Never users' of oral contraceptives the Spearman r_S between breast size and body mass index (BMI) is + 0.47.

Only BMI and weight are significantly associated with breast size among this group (p-values <0.05).

Breast size is not significantly associated with any of the variables among current oral contraceptive users (all p-values ≥ 0.05).

TABLE 6. Spearman rank correlations (r_S) between breast sizes in healthy Swedish female university students, according to oral contraceptive use and body mass index, height, weight, family history of breast cancer, age at menarche, and age, 1993–1994*

| | Oral contraceptive use | | | | | | | |
| | Never users (n=20) | | Former users (n=20) | | All nonusers (n=40) | | Current users (n=25) | |
	r_S	p	r_S	p	r_S	p	r_S	p
Body mass index[†]	0.47	0.038	0.71	<0.001	0.53	<0.001	0.27	0.196
Height	0.25	0.286	0.42	0.068	0.32	0.046	−0.06	0.783
Weight	0.47	0.037	0.55	0.011	0.50	0.001	0.24	0.248
Family history of breast cancer in a first or second degree relative	−0.17	0.473	−0.41	0.071	−0.24	0.131	0.01	0.951
Age at menarche	−0.23	0.329	0.03	0.889	−0.06	0.735	−0.08	0.707
Waist:hip ratio	−0.00	0.985	0.35	0.133	0.18	0.256	0.25	0.226
Age	0.09	0.718	−0.20	0.396	−0.04	0.814	0.15	0.480

* Values from measurements taken during menstrual cycle days 5–10 were used.
[†] Weight (kg)/height (m)^2.

FIGURE 22.5 Spearman correlation coefficients between breast size and a number of factors, according to oral contraceptive use

used Spearman's r_S to measure association, perhaps because of doubts about the Normality of the variables, or the accuracy of recalled data. Their results are shown in Figure 22.5. The authors have chosen to use p-values rather than confidence intervals to test the significance of the r_S values.

Figure 22.5 shows that, apart from body mass index among non-oral contraceptive users, breast size appears to have no connection with most of these physical measurements. It is not surprising that *weight* has an association if BMI does since the two are linearly related through the formula for BMI (as noted in the table footnote). But again it's not clear which correlation coefficient has been used for the association between breast size and the family history of breast cancer variable, which is dichotomous (yes/no), and for which Spearman's r_S is not suitable.

Correlation implies nothing about *causality*, i.e. about whether there is a *relationship* (as opposed to simply an association) between any two variables. That is, do changes in one variable bring about or *cause* changes in the other variable, and if so, in what way? To answer these questions we need multivariable methods which we will come to in Chapter 24.

We noted at the beginning of this chapter that association and agreement measure two different things. Association measures the degree to which two sets of values tend to move *together*. Agreement measures the degree to which the values are actually the *same*. However, even if two variables are *associated*, they may not *agree* very well (although if two variables agree they will clearly be associated). Spearmans' r_S for the Glasgow Coma Scale scores given in the example at the beginning of this chapter was +0.962 with a 95% CI of (0.844 to 0.991). So the association between the scores is strong. However, the percentage of scores which *agree* is only 20% (2 in 10), so agreement is poor.

Whenever you read a paper containing correlation calculations, you should be able to tell which correlation coefficient has been used for which data. We can now turn to the methods used by authors to measure agreement.

23

Measuring Agreement

In Chapter 22 we looked at methods used by authors to measure the level of *association* between two variables, and we noted in passing that association and agreement are not the same. We now want to describe how authors report the degree of *agreement* between two variables. As usual the type of data involved influences the choice of measure (see Chapter 11). We'll start with nominal data and the use of *kappa*. We have already encountered the use of kappa to measure agreement by means of test–retest reliability (see Chapter 15 on measurement scales).

NOMINAL DATA: KAPPA

Suppose you asked two GPs to examine separately 10 patients and state whether or not they had a particular medical condition. They produced the following results:

Patient	1	2	3	4	5	6	7	8	9	10
GP A	Y	Y	Y	N	Y	N	N	Y	Y	N
GP B	N	Y	Y	Y	Y	N	N	N	Y	Y

The GPs agreed with each other on six patients but disagreed on four. So their *observed proportional agreement* was $6/10 = 0.6$. However, we would have expected them to agree by chance on a few of them anyway, even if they had to take a wild guess without even seeing the patients. What we need is a measure which adjusts the observed agreement for the number of agreements which are due to chance alone. This is what *kappa* (written as κ) does. Kappa measures the proportion of scores which agree (i.e. fall in the same category) *adjusted* for the proportion which could be expected to agree by chance. Kappa is properly known as the *chance-corrected proportional agreement statistic*.

Interpreting κ

Kappa can vary between 0 (no agreement) and 1 (perfect agreement). Values of kappa may be assessed with the help of Table 23.1. Only values for kappa of about 0.60 or more indicate good agreement. In general, variables which are found to be firmly *associated* will usually show good *agreement*, and vice versa, although, since this is not invariably the case, the methods are not interchangeable.

One weakness of kappa is that it is sensitive to the proportion of subjects in each category, in other words, prevalence. The consequence of this is that kappas from different studies should not be compared if the prevalences are not the same. Kappa has many applications, and two typical examples are given below.

Figure 23.1 is taken from a study exploring differences in agreement on their sexual behaviour in the past 12 months, between Thai couples, according to their respective HIV status. In one group both partners were HIV+, in the other group only one of the partners was. The figure shows the levels of both of the couples total % observed agreement and of their chance-corrected (kappa) agreement. As you can

Understanding Clinical Papers Second Edition   David Bowers, Allan House, David Owens

TABLE 23.1   Assessing agreement with kappa

κ	Strength of agreement
<0.20	Poor
0.21–0.40	Fair
0.41–0.60	Moderate
0.61–0.80	Good
0.81–1.00	Very good

see, although total observed % agreement between the groups was quite similar, overall chance-corrected agreement was quite different.

Figure 23.2 is from a study into the effects of passive smoking on coronary heart disease. The authors used kappa to test the *reliability* of data on exposure to risk factors as reported by the subjects in the study. From the original sample of 185, 35 subjects were re-interviewed and their responses were

Reliability of Self-Reported Sexual Behaviour in Human Immunodeficiency Virus (HIV) Between Concordant and Discordant Heterosexual Couples in Northern Thailand

Melanie A. de Boer, David D. Celentano, Sodsai Tovanabutra, Sungwal Rugpao, Kenrad E. Nelson, and Vinai Suriyanon

Where both partners are HIV+, oral sex taking place in past year is reported by 24 males but 33 females, ...

... giving an observed agreement of 76%, but a chance adjusted agreement of only κ = 0.10 (poor), ...

... whereas when only one partner is HIV+, there is a similar, 77 %, observed agreement on oral sex happening but chance-adjusted agreement has improved, κ = 0.27 (fair).

Sexual behaviour	Both partners HIV+ (n=246)			Only one partner HIV+ (n=283)		
	No. positive reports (male/female)	% observed agreement	Kappa	No. positive reports (male/female)	% observed agreement	Kappa
Vaginal sex	246/246	100	?	283/283	100	?
Oral sex	24/33	76	0.10	34/49	77	0.27
Anal sex	6/4	96	0.16	13/8	93	0.06
No condom use in last 2 years	104/88	78	0.54	122/104	82	0.65
Condom use > 50% of time in past year	30/26	90	0.50	36/26	91	0.25

FIGURE 23.1   Agreement between partners of sexual behaviour in the past year, by HIV status

Passive smoking at work as a risk factor for coronary heart disease in Chinese women who have never smoked

Y He, T H Lam, L S Li, R Y Du, G L Jia, J Y Huang, J S Zheng

Results on single blind test-re-test by two interviewers on 35 hospital subjects (16 cases and 19 controls) showed good agreement, ranging from 75% to 95% for the 10 risk factors tested, with κ values ranging from 0.4 to 0.8 (nine κ values with P<0.01 and one with P<0.05; data not shown).

In this example kappa is used to test the reliability of patient-recorded data, by re-interviewing a subsample of the original sample. This is the test–retest procedure.

FIGURE 23.2   Extract from a passive smoking study with the authors' description of using kappa for measuring agreement in a test–retest

compared with their original responses (this procedure is known as *test–retest*). Kappa was used to measure the level of agreement between first and second interviews.

Values for kappa are also shown in Figure 22.4 from the study on the medical record validation of maternally reported birth characteristics. Generally speaking, the higher values of kappa are associated with the higher correlation coefficient values, and vice versa, but not entirely consistently.

ORDINAL DATA: WEIGHTED KAPPA

If the categories can be *ordered* (for example, ordinal scores, discrete metric, or grouped metric scores), then researchers can calculate a version of kappa which is adjusted (or *weighted*) to allow for 'near misses'. This idea is best illustrated with an example. Two experienced trauma doctors were asked to rate 16 patients using the Injury Severity Score (ISS), a scale for assessing the severity of trauma (ISS varies from 0 to 75). The data are shown in Table 23.2. The doctors agree on only 5 out of 16 cases, so the level of exact agreement is low.

However, in several cases the scores although not identical are close (for example, patients 2 and 6), whereas in other cases they are further apart (for example, patients 9 and 15). Weighted kappa gives credit to those scores which although not exactly in agreement are at least close, and less credit to those further apart. The frequency with which weighted kappa appears in clinical papers does not justify any further discussion here.

TABLE 23.2   Injury Severity Scale scores given by two observers to 16 trauma patients

	Patients															
Doctors	1	2	3	4	5	6	7	8	9	10	11	12	13	14	15	16
1	9	14	29	17	34	17	38	29	4	29	25	4	16	25	25	45
2	9	13	29	17	22	14	45	10	29	4	25	34	9	25	8	50

METRIC DATA

Unfortunately there is no single statistic which researchers can use to report agreement between two metric variables. Kappa is of little use since the large number of possible values means that there will be few, if any, pairs of values which are exactly the same. And as we have seen, correlation does not do the same job. One method has been suggested by Bland & Altman (1986). This involves plotting the *differences* between each pair of scores (vertical axis) against their mean (horizontal axis).

In this plot, points showing perfect agreement will lie exactly on the horizontal line drawn through the value 0. The further away the points lie from this line, the worse the level of agreement. Moreover the points should be scattered more or less horizontally – an indication that the level of agreement is approximately the same over the whole range of values.

One way of assessing the acceptability of the agreement level is to calculate the standard deviation of the difference scores and then draw two horizontal lines at plus and minus two times this standard deviation. If most of the points lie within these tramlines, then agreement between the two measures may be deemed acceptable.

As an example of the Bland–Altman procedure, Figure 23.3 is from a study to assess the accuracy and reliability of two non-invasive thermometers: a chemical thermometer, and a tympanic thermometer, by comparing them to the gold-standard pulmonary artery catheter (PAC). Temperature data are metric and the authors show two Bland–Altman plots to measure agreement between the PAC and the chemical and tympanic thermometers respectively. The authors have added the ± 2 s.d. tramlines.

As you can see, the agreement of the PAC with the chemical thermometer is slightly biased by $+0.2°C$ (chemical thermometer measuring $+0.2$ °C more than the PAC), but overall agreement is closer, 2s.d.s $= 0.7°C$, compared to the tympanic thermometer's 2s.d.s $= 1.2°C$, although the latter is unbiased. There is no evidence that agreement deteriorates over the range of either instrument.

We promised towards the end of Chapter 22 that we would need to turn to methods of analysis, other than association, which authors use to investigate causal relationship between variables. In Chapter 24 we do so.

Temperature measurement: comparison of non-invasive methods used in adult critical care

Sarah Farnell, Loraine Maxwell, Seok Tan, Andrew Rhodes, and Barbara Philips

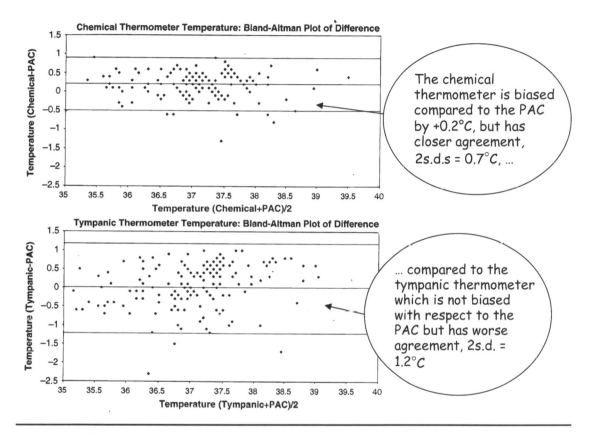

FIGURE 23.3 Use of the Bland–Altman plot to compare two thermometers, chemical and tympanic with the gold standard pulmonary artery catheter (PAC)

24

The Linear Regression Model

WHY REGRESSION?

The ideas examined in this chapter are a little more complex than some of the other material in this book. Unfortunately, to understand journal papers which present the results of the sorts of analysis discussed below, and to point out what you as a reader need to look out for, we must spend at least a little time discussing some of the basic ideas. We have, as usual, tried to avoid being too technical.

We noted at the end of Chapter 21 that association does not imply causation. If we were to examine the association between smoking and coronary heart disease (CHD), we would no doubt find that the two measures were significantly positively correlated; in general, the more people smoke, the greater their likelihood of coronary heart disease, and vice versa. But this association does not *necessarily* mean that it is smoking which *causes* CHD, nor that having CHD *causes* people to smoke. We can only say that the two are associated.

Similarly, the chi-squared test will tell us whether two categorical variables are independent or not, but *only* two variables and they have to be categorical (or metric variables which can be categorized). Moreover, the chi-squared test is *only* a test, it does not indicate anything about the nature of the relationship (if one exists), i.e. the existence or direction of causality, or any size effects. So both correlation and chi-squared, although useful procedures, have limitations.

In practice, of course, if researchers suspect a causal relationship between one variable and another (more usually, several others), they will also have a belief about the direction of that relationship (smoking causes CHD). To investigate such relationships they can turn to a powerful class of modelling procedures, collectively known as *multivariable analysis*, within which *regression analysis* is perhaps the most widely used. In the next three chapters we want to discuss three different types of regression: linear regression (in this chapter), logistic regression (Chapter 25), and proportional (or Cox) regression (Chapter 27 in the context of survival analysis). We must also give a passing mention to *analysis of variance*, related to regression, as you will see, and popular in psychology.

LINEAR REGRESSION

To state the blindingly obvious, regression analysis is done with a regression model, a mathematical equation which captures the nature and direction of a causal relationship between one variable and one or more other variables. We'll begin with the *linear regression model*, since this is the easiest to explain.

To illustrate the general idea, suppose your favourite clinic pastime is to guess each patient's systolic blood pressure (SBP), before it is measured. To your colleagues' surprise, you are quite good at it, but they don't know that its all down to a bit of mental arithmetic (but based on having seen a lot of patients). Here's how you do it. For every patient, you always start with the number 4, to which you add

Understanding Clinical Papers Second Edition   David Bowers, Allan House, David Owens
© 2006 John Wiley & Sons, Ltd

their age (which you know from their record) multiplied by one and a half; then add their hip girth in cm (which you've grown very good at estimating by eye) multiplied by a third; then add 10 if they are male; and a further 10 if they are smokers (which you also know from the record). Let's write your mental sum as an equation:

$$\text{Systolic blood pressure(mmHg)} = 4 + (1.5 \times \text{age}) + (0.333 \times \text{hip girth}) + (10 \times \text{sex}) + (10 \times \text{smoker})$$

where *sex* will equal 0 if female and 1 if male, and *smoker* will equal 0 if a non-smoker and 1 if a smoker.

To illustrate, if the next patient is a 50-year-old non-smoking male, with a hip girth of 240 cm, then you would estimate his systolic blood pressure to be:

$$\text{SBP} = 4 + (1.5 \times 50) + (0.333 \times 240) + (10 \times 1) + (10 \times 0)$$
$$= 149 \, \text{mmHg}$$

And this is a *multivariable linear regression model*. The model is said to be multivariable because there is more than one variable on the right-hand side of the equation, namely, *age, hip girth, sex* and *smoker*. These right-hand-side variables are called the *independent, explanatory*, or *predictor* variables, or just the *covariates*. These may be metric, ordinal or nominal, and don't have to be Normally distributed. The variable to the left of the = sign (systolic blood pressure in this example) is called the *dependent, outcome* or *response* variable, and *must* be metric continuous.

Finally, the model is said to be *linear* because we assume that the effect on systolic blood pressure of an increase in age, say, from 50 to 51, is the same as for age increases from 90 to 91 or 20 to 21 or any other one-year increase. In other words, the effect of a change in age on systolic blood pressure remains the same right across the age range, and if we were to plot systolic blood pressure against age we would observe that the points were scattered evenly around a straight line, as we saw in Figure 22.1. And this needs also to be true for each of the other independent variables.

Clearly for some variables this linearity assumption will not be appropriate and authors should provide clear evidence that they have tested for it, something you should be able to readily confirm from the paper (we'll see how authors can do this shortly).

In practice, we should add an uncertainty term (called the *error* or *residual* term) to the above equation. However good you are at this guessing game, you can never account for random variations, and so you are never likely to be spot on (except coincidentally). So the residual term accounts for the difference between your guess of systolic blood pressure and its true value. If we label the residual as *e* and abbreviate the other variable names, we can summarize the main components of the linear regression model as in Figure 24.1.

The value and sign of each coefficient give us an *estimate* of the magnitude and direction of the change in the dependent variable if the corresponding independent variable increases by one unit. For example, in our systolic blood pressure model, if age increases by one year (age is measured in units of one year) then systolic blood pressure will also *increase* (because the sign of the age coefficient, 1.5, is *positive*) by 1.5 mmHg. The single number on its own (4) is called the constant coefficient or just the *constant*, and is usually ignored. The only role it plays is to keep an arithmetic balance between the left- and right-hand sides of the regression equation.

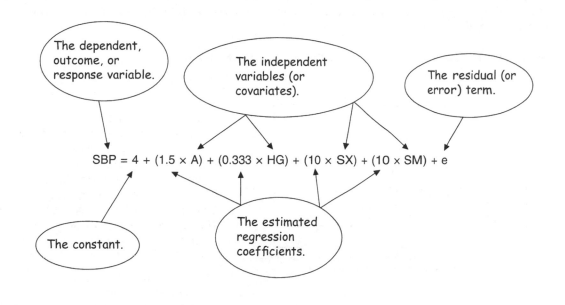

FIGURE **24.1**   The main components of a linear regression model

In more general terms, the multiple linear regression equation is written as:

$$Y = \beta_0 + \beta_1 \times X_1 + \beta_2 \times X_2 + \cdots + e$$

where β_1, β_2, etc., are called the *population regression coefficients*.

The Regression Coefficients – Ordinary Least Squares Estimation

In our systolic blood pressure equation above, the number in front of each variable (1.5, 0.333, 10 and 10), are called the *sample regression coefficients*. They are our estimates of the population regression coefficients β_1, β_2, and so on. In practice, of course, these values have to be estimated from the sample data, rather than being simply guessed!

Authors will not usually refer to the estimation process they use, but almost invariably it will be the method of *ordinary least squares* or OLS (although some computer programs use what is called maximum likelihood estimation). Briefly put, OLS minimizes the sum of all the squared error terms (Σe^2). The regression line which is produced by this method gives the 'best' estimates of the population regression coefficients (i.e. at least as close to the true population coefficient values as any other method). The idea is illustrated in Figure 24.2. This shows a regression line drawn through a scatter plot of birthweight against cord serum EPA concentration.

Birthweight in a fishing community: significance of essential fatty acids and marine food contaminants

Philippe Grandjean, Kristian S Bjerve, Pál Weihe and Ulrike Steuerwald

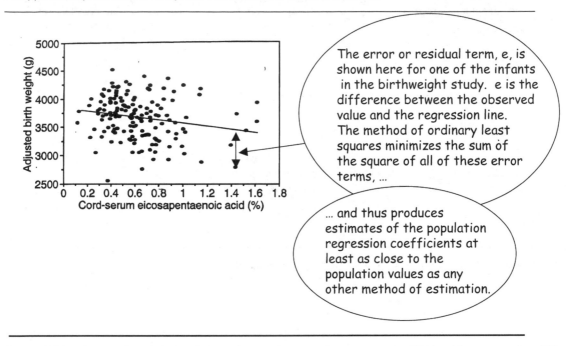

FIGURE 24.2   Scatter plot of birthweight against cord serum eicosapentaenoic (EPA) acid concentration. EPA concentration is a measure of the availability of polyunsaturated fatty acids to the foetus, and is thought to influence foetal growth

MEASURING THE STATISTICAL SIGNIFICANCE OF THE REGRESSION PARAMETERS

Since the sample regression coefficients (such as 1.5, 0.333, 10, and 10, in our blood pressure example above) are only *estimates* of the true population parameter values, β_1, β_2, etc., we need to know whether or not they are statistically significant. In this case, are they significantly different from 0? Obviously, if a population regression coefficient is zero, the independent variable with which it is associated cannot possibly have *any* influence on the dependent variable – it doesn't matter what value this variable takes, once its multiplied by 0, it drops out. Of course, even if a population coefficient *is* zero, it doesn't mean (samples being what they are) that its *sample* coefficient will be zero (and in practice it *never* is). That's why researchers need to assess the statistical significance of each coefficient.

You won't be surprised to learn that they do this either by calculating a confidence interval for each sample coefficient (does it contain 0?) or a *p*-value (is it less than 0.05?), or less frequently its standard error, SE. See Chapters 19 and 21 if you need a reminder. In other words: for each regression coefficient, if either the *p*-value is less than 0.05, or the 95% confidence interval does *not* contain 0, then that coefficient's variable has a significant influence on the dependent variable in the population. The standard error is less useful, but as a rule of thumb, if a coefficient divided by its standard error is >2, then the coefficient is significantly different from 0.

So when you read a paper which uses linear regression you should be able to find either the p-value for each coefficient, or better, a confidence interval, in the table of results. By the way, establishing significance in a regression model does not prove causality. The causal nature of a relationship (if any) depends on the inherent nature of the variables.

MODEL BUILDING AND VARIABLE SELECTION

At the beginning of this chapter we assumed that you knew which variables you needed to use to predict the systolic blood pressure of your patients. In practice, researchers may or may not have a working hypothesis about the variables they think will play a role in explaining the variation in their outcome variable. Whether they do or don't will influence their variable selection procedure, i.e. how they build their regression model. Authors may refer to their choice of model building procedure so we need to say a few words about the possibilities.

There are two main approaches. First, automated variable selection – the computer does it for you. This approach is perhaps more appropriate if you have little idea about which variables are likely to be relevant in the relationship. A second possibility is manual selection – you do it! This approach is more appropriate if you have a particular hypothesis to test, so that you have a pretty good idea which explanatory variable is likely to be the most interesting in explaining your outcome variable, but you may want to control for other potentially confounding, variables (see p. 58 for an account of confounding).

What follows is a very brief description of some of the variable selection procedures, starting with automated methods first. Note that the criteria used by the various computer regression programs to select and de-select variables vary from program to program. Most of these methods start with a series of *univariate* regressions, i.e. each explanatory variable in turn is regressed against the outcome variable and the p-value noted. At this stage all variables which have a p-value ≤ 0.2 or thereabouts should be considered as candidate variables – using a p-value less than this may fail to identify variables which could turn out to be important in the final model.

Automated Variable Selection Methods

- *Forwards selection*: The computer program starts with the variable which has the lowest p-value (from the univariate regressions). It then adds the other variables one at a time, in lowest p-value order, until all variables with p-values <0.05 are included.
- *Backwards selection*: The reverse of forwards selection. The program starts with all of the candidate variables included in the model, then the variable which has highest p-value >0.05, is removed. Then the next highest p-value variable, and so on, until only those variables with a p-value <0.05 are left in the model and all other variables have been discarded.
- *Forward or backward stepwise selection*: After each variable is added (or removed), the variables which were already (or are left) in the model are re-checked for statistical significance; if no longer significant they are removed. The end result is a model where all variables have a p-value <0.05.

These automated procedures have a number of potential disadvantages, (including misleadingly narrow confidence intervals and exaggeration of coefficient values, and thus their effect size), although they may be useful when researchers have little idea about which variables are likely to be relevant. As an example of this approach the authors of a study into the role of arginase in sickle cell disease, in which the outcome variable was $\log_{10}$ arginase activity (transformed because of distributional problems), comment:

This modelling used a stepwise procedure to add independent variables, beginning with the variables most strongly associated with $\log_{10}$ arginase with $P \leq 0.15$. Deletion of variables after initial inclusion in the model was allowed. The procedure continued until all independent variables in the final model had $P \leq 0.05$, adjusted for other independent variables, and no additional variables had $P \leq 0.05$.

Manual Variable Selection Methods

These methods are often more appropriate if the investigators are trying to explore the relationship between two variables, say between birthweight and length of gestation period, and wish to *adjust* for any possible confounding variables, such as sex of baby, smoking during pregnancy, mother's weight, and so on. The identity of potential confounders will have been established by experience, a literature search, discussions with colleagues and patients, and so on. There are two alternative manual selection procedures.

- *Backward elimination*: The main variable plus all of the potentially confounding variables are entered into the model at the start. The results will then reveal which variables are statistically significant (*p*-value <0.05). Non-significant variables can then be dropped, one at a time in decreasing *p*-value order, from the model, unless the coefficient of any of the remaining variables changes markedly when a variable is dropped, in which case the variable should be retained since this may indicate that it is a confounder. (These is no rule about how big a change in a coefficient should be considered noteworthy. A value of 10% has been suggested, but this seems on the small side.)
- *Forward elimination*: The main variable of interest is put in the model, and the other (confounding) variables are added one at a time in order of (lowest) *p*-value (from the univariate regressions). If statistically significant they are retained, if not, they are dropped, unless any of the coefficients of the existing variables change noticeably suggesting that the new variable may be a confounder.

The end result of either manual approach should be a model containing the same variables (although this model may differ from a model derived using one of the automated procedures). In any case, the overall objective is *parsimony*, i.e. having as few explanatory variables in the model as possible while at the same time explaining the maximum amount of variation in the outcome variable. Parsimony is particularly important when sample size is on the small side; as a rule of thumb, researchers will need at least 20 observations for each independent variable to obtain reasonable statistical reliability (e.g. narrow-ish confidence intervals).

As an example of the manual backwards selection approach, the authors of the birthweight and cord serum EPA concentration (Figure 24.2) knew that cord serum EPA was their principal explanatory variable, and only wanted to add possible confounders to their model. They commented:

> Multiple regression analysis was used to determine the relevant importance of predictors of the outcome (variable). Potential confounders were identified on the basis of previous studies, and included maternal height and weight, smoking during pregnancy, diabetes, parity, gestational length, and sex of the child. Covariates were kept in the final regression equation if statistically significant ($p < 0.01$) after backwards elimination.

Incidentally, the main explanatory variable, cord serum concentration, was found to be statistically significant (*p*-value $= 0.037$), as were all of the confounding variables.

Adjustment

One important feature of regression models makes them very attractive to researchers. The effect that each explanatory variable has on the dependent variable (as expressed by its coefficient value) is *adjusted* to discount any possible interactions with the other independent variables. In effect, any possible influence of the other independent variables in the model is *controlled for.*

A coefficient thus measures only the *'pure'* effect on the dependent variable of a change by one unit in its own independent variable. This result is hard to achieve using alternative methods of analysis. As we have seen, one further major advantage of this is that it enables the effects of potential *confounding variables* to be examined. Before we discuss confounding, let's look at the first example below.

Figure 24.3 is from a study into the effect of chronic hypertension in women on the risk of small-for-gestational-age babies, in which the dependent variable is *birthweight* (g) adjusted for gestational age at delivery. The explanatory variable of principal focus is chronic hypertension, but a number of other variables are included since the authors believed that they needed to be adjusted for. These include smoking, and mother's weight, height, age, parity, ethnic origin and educational level. These other variables are a mix of metric, ordinal and nominal types. Figure 24.3 shows, for each independent variable, its estimated coefficient value, generally denoted 'β', the standard error SE (a measure of the preciseness of the estimate – smaller is better), and the *p*-value.

Effect of Uncomplicated Chronic Hypertension on the Risk of Small-for-Gestational Age Birth

Edwige Haelterman,[1] Gérard Bréart,[2] Josefa Paris-Llado,[2] Michèle Dramaix,[1] and Catherine Tchobroutsky[2,3]

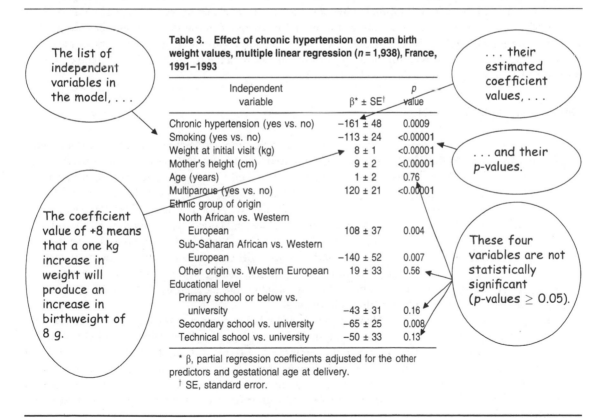

Table 3. Effect of chronic hypertension on mean birth weight values, multiple linear regression (*n* = 1,938), France, 1991–1993

Independent variable	$\beta^* \pm SE^\dagger$	*p* value
Chronic hypertension (yes vs. no)	−161 ± 48	0.0009
Smoking (yes vs. no)	−113 ± 24	<0.00001
Weight at initial visit (kg)	8 ± 1	<0.00001
Mother's height (cm)	9 ± 2	<0.00001
Age (years)	1 ± 2	0.76
Multiparous (yes vs. no)	120 ± 21	<0.00001
Ethnic group of origin		
North African vs. Western European	108 ± 37	0.004
Sub-Saharan African vs. Western European	−140 ± 52	0.007
Other origin vs. Western European	19 ± 33	0.56
Educational level		
Primary school or below vs. university	−43 ± 31	0.16
Secondary school vs. university	−65 ± 25	0.008
Technical school vs. university	−50 ± 33	0.13

* β, partial regression coefficients adjusted for the other predictors and gestational age at delivery.
$\dagger$ SE, standard error.

The list of independent variables in the model, . . .

. . . their estimated coefficient values, . . .

. . . and their p-values.

The coefficient value of +8 means that a one kg increase in weight will produce an increase in birthweight of 8 g.

These four variables are not statistically significant (p-values ≥ 0.05).

FIGURE 24.3   Results of multiple linear regression analysis of chronic hypertension on risk of small babies

We can see that most of the explanatory variables are significant contributors to birthweight. The exceptions are: mother's *Age* (*p*-value $= 0.76$); *Other ethnic origin vs. Western European* (*p*-value $= 0.56$); and two of the *Educational level* variables (*p*-values $= 0.16$ and 0.13). In particular, chronic hypertension, the focus of the study, is a statistically significant factor in low-birthweight babies (*p*-value $= 0.0009$).

Interpreting the Regression Coefficients

We explained earlier that the value of the regression coefficient tells us by how much the outcome variable changes if the explanatory variable increases by 1 unit of measurement. For example, in the hypertensive study, the value of the coefficient of $+8$ for the variable 'Mothers weight at initial visit' means that for every unit increase in mothers weight by 1 kg, birthweight increases by an average of 8 g. The value for the chronic hypertension coefficient of -161 means that for every unit increase in hypertension, i.e. from 0 (no hypertension) to 1 (hypertension), birthweight *decreases* by an average of 161 g. Finally, if a mother has an educational level of primary school or below compared to a university-educated mother, then birthweight will be 43 g lower on average.

Goodness of Fit

Authors may also report a *goodness-of-fit statistic* R^2 (also known as the coefficient of determination), which you may see quoted. R^2, which can vary between 0 and 1, measures the proportion of the variation in the outcome variable which is *explained* by the collection of explanatory variables. The value of R^2 is thus used as an indication of the quality of the model in terms of fitting the data, and can be used to compare alternative models. Note, however, that when you add a variable to an existing model and you want to compare the goodness-of-fit of the augmented model with the original model, you have to use a variant of R^2 known as *adjusted* R^2, and denoted $\overline{R}^2$.

Dummy (or Design) Variables

As you have seen, linear regression models may contain *nominal* explanatory variables, for example, 'Ethnic origin' as in Figure 24.3. This variable has four categories: European, North African, Sub-Saharan African, and Other. These categories have to be given numerical values before they can be entered into the computer regression program, but they cannot simply be allocated the numbers 1, 2, 3 and 4, since the four categories have no meaningful ordering – why not 3, 4, 1, 2? Instead, the categories have to be represented by a set of design or *dummy* variables and coded appropriately, and the original variable, ethnicity in our example, replaced by these dummies. Since authors commonly use dummy variables we need to say a few words about them. As you will see, we need one less dummy variable than there are categories in the original variable. A simple coding scheme, such as that shown in Table 24.1 is commonly used. Here the three dummy variables are labelled E1, E2 and E3, and applied to the Ethnic origin variable in the birthweight example.

So instead of the original single 'Ethnic origin' variable being entered into the model (which it can't be with any meaningful values), the three dummy variables take its place. Thus an individual who's ethnic origin is Sub-Saharan Africa is given the values: E1 $= 0$, E2 $= 1$ and E3 $= 0$ in the data. Most computer programs will allow you to choose a *reference* or referent category. In this example the authors have chosen 'European' as their reference category, so that for example, the coefficient on Sub-Saharan African which has a value of -140 (see Figure 24.3) is with reference to the birthweight of infants with ethnically European mothers.

Table **24.1** A simple coding design for the nominal variable 'Ethic origin' in a study of birthweight (see Figure 24.3)

Ethnic category	Dummy variable		
	E1	E2	E3
European	0	0	0
North African	0	0	1
Sub-Saharan African	0	1	0
Other	1	0	0

Use of three dummy variables to code the four-category ethnic origin variable in Figure 23.2. The 'European' category is the reference category. We will always need one less dummy variable than the number of categories in the variable in question.

Binary nominal variables, the most common example being sex, are also coded with a dummy variable, i.e. the two categories, male and female, are replaced with one dummy variable which can take the value 0 (for a male, say) or 1 (for a female). We do this without thinking!

If authors include nominal variables with more than two categories in a regression model, they should explain their coding design, and indicate clearly their reference category. Ordinal and metric variables can be entered into the model 'as is', i.e. without the need for coding (unless there is *strong* clinical evidence to suggest that the relationship may be non-linear).

Testing the Assumptions of the Linear Regression Model

We have already seen that the outcome variable must be metric and that the relationship between the outcome variable and the explanatory or independent variable(s) has to be linear, if we are to use linear regression analysis. There are a few more conditions which must also be met. The more complete list is as follows:

- The outcome (or dependent) variable must be metric.
- The relationship between the outcome variable and the independent variable(s) must be linear.
- The error term e must be Normally distributed with a mean of 0 for each value of each explanatory variable.
- The spread of the error term must be the same for each value of each explanatory variable (this the property known as *homoskedasticity*).
- None of the explanatory variables should be perfectly correlated with any other of the explanatory variables (if this condition is not satisfied, then the model is said to suffer from *multicollinearity*). Most models will suffer from some degree of collinearity among the explanatory variable set.

Authors will not usually refer to these conditions specifically but should provide some evidence that they have checked that at least the linearity of the relationship, and the Normalness and constant spread of the error term conditions are satisfied. Only when these conditions are met will the method of ordinary least squares produce the best estimates of the population coefficients.

The first condition is or is not self-evident (although many journal papers contain linear regression results with an ordinal outcome variable!). The second condition of linearity is usually assumed and rarely examined. The third and fourth conditions relating to the error term are sometimes tested. The last condition of no collinearity between the explanatory variables is infrequently tested but obvious pitfalls should be avoided, e.g. having both diastolic and systolic blood pressure, in a model – these are almost certain to be correlated.

Figure 24.4 shows the sorts of plot which you might expect to see (or at least see referred to). Figure 24.4(a) is a scatter which indicates that all three assumptions are met. Figure 24.4(b) shows a scatter which indicates a non-constant spread – as the values of the independent variable increase, so does the spread of the error terms. Figure 24.4(c) shows that the relationship is not linear, nor is the spread constant.

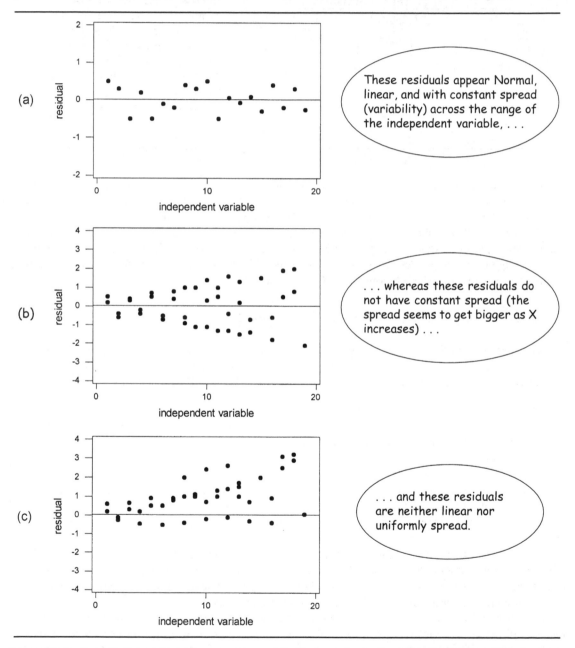

FIGURE 24.4 Examination of the basic assumptions of the linear regression model by plotting the residuals against values of each independent variable in turn. The scatter should be broadly horizontal and of uniform spread across the range of each independent variable

Association between child and adolescent television viewing and adult health: a longitudinal birth cohort study

Robert J Hancox, Barry J Milne, Richard Poulton

We checked linear regression models by visual inspection of the residuals (error terms) to ensure that they were normal in distribution and that they were randomly scattered versus the fitted values.

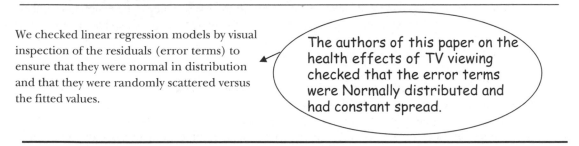

The authors of this paper on the health effects of TV viewing checked that the error terms were Normally distributed and had constant spread.

FIGURE 24.5 Checking the properties of the error or residual term

As an alternative to plotting the residuals against each independent variable, researchers can use either a *statistical test* of Normality, or produce a *Normal plot* of the residuals. Both of these possibilities are available in all good statistical programs. Space prevents any further consideration of these options. Nonetheless, it should be possible for you to find some evidence that the authors have examined the assumptions referred to above, although in practice such evidence is only infrequently provided.

As an example from practice, Figure 24.5 contains an extract from a study of the association between child television viewing and adult health. The authors report testing the error term assumptions but provided no graphical evidence that the basic conditions were satisfied.

Effect Modification and Interaction

Suppose we are using a linear regression model to investigate the relationship between systolic blood pressure (the dependent variable) and age, among a group of individuals, and we have included gender as a possible confounder. If we discover that systolic blood pressure is related to age but the relationship is significantly different for men and women, then we would say that systolic blood pressure and gender are *interacting*. We call gender an *effect modifier* because it is acting to modify the effect of age on systolic blood pressure according to whether the individual is a male or female. If gender was only a confounder and not an effect modifier, it would affect the relationship between age and systolic blood pressure equally for both men and women. So effect modification differs from confounding in that the latter is present for all sub-groups and at all levels, whereas an effect modifier acts differentially at different levels and/or with different subgroups.

The presence of effect modification can be tested by including an interaction term as an additional independent variable in the model. This term will usually be formed from the product of the two variables in question, in this case (gender × age). If it turns out to have a *p*-value <0.05, this suggests that effect modification might be present. Authors should only introduce an interaction term in their model if they have made a *strong* case for its inclusion on clinical grounds, and should not be included if no *main* effect has been found to be statistically significant. The introduction of interaction terms diminishes the model's parsimony (especially if it involves multiple terms in a dummy variable), and may thus lead to problems with sample size.

Summary

The linear regression model is an extremely useful tool for investigating the nature of a possible relationship between some outcome (or dependent) variable and several explanatory (or independent) variables, particularly since it allows researchers to adjust for confounders, something difficult to achieve with any other method. When you are reading a clinical paper which reports on the use of a linear regression model, there are, as you have seen, many things to take in. However, at a minimum, the authors should do the following:

- Justify the linear nature of the relationship.
- Provide a list of candidate variables.
- Explain their variable selection procedure (forward, backward, manual, etc.).
- Provide a list of the variables in the final model.
- Explain the coding system for any dummy variables included in the model.
- Present values for the estimated coefficients, preferably with confidence intervals rather than (or as well as) p-values.
- Offer a reasonably detailed interpretation of their results.
- Say something about the goodness-of-fit of their model, i.e. by quoting R^2.
- Test the basic assumptions (is the error term Normally distributed with constant spread?)

Although the linear regression model frequently appears in clinical papers, the logistic regression model is perhaps even more ubiquitous. We will discuss this procedure in Chapter 25.

ANALYSIS OF VARIANCE

The results of a procedure known as analysis of variance or *Anova*, sometimes appears in clinical papers, so needs a brief mention. Linear regression and Anova can be shown to be identical facets of what is known to mathematicians as the *generalized linear model*. Anova has a history in the social sciences, particularly psychology and related fields.

However, everything that Anova can do, regression can do, and seems to us to be easier to understand. Andy Field (2000) in his book on statistics and SPSS, says:

> Anova (known as the variance-ratio method) is fine for simple designs, but becomes impossibly cumbersome in more complex situations. The regression model extends very logically to these more complex designs ... without getting bogged down in mathematics. Finally, ... the method becomes extremely unmanageable in some circumstances, such as unequal sample sizes. The regression method makes these situations considerably more simple.

Because Anova is not frequently encountered in the principal clinical journals, and because of space limitations, we will not consider it further in this book. Those who want to learn more could do worse than refer to Andy Field's book, or to Altman (1991).

MULTIVARIATE STATISTICS

There is another powerful class of statistical procedures known collectively as *multivariate statistics*. The multivariate approach is appropriate when there is more than one outcome variable. Included among these methods are factor analysis, discriminant analysis, and multidimensional scaling. Although these ideas can be very versatile, they are not seen in the journals with enough frequency to justify any space being devoted to them here.

25

The Logistic Regression Model

In the multiple linear regression model considered in Chapter 24, the outcome variable, systolic blood pressure, was a continuous variable. However, clinical researchers often work with binary outcome variables, i.e. those which can take only two values (alive or dead, relapsed or didn't relapse, malignant or benign, etc.). These two possibilities are usually coded 0 and 1. In these circumstances *logistic regression* models are appropriate. Logistic regression is popular because it provides values for the *odds, risk* and *hazard* ratios (see Chapter 18) for any independent variables which are considered to affect (adversely or beneficially) the outcome variable. Such independent variables are often known as *risk factors*. Logistic regression *can* be used with outcome variables which have more than two possible values, known as ordinal logistic regression although these appear rarely and will not be discussed here.

THE MODEL

Although you won't see the mathematical form of the binary logistic model appearing in clinical papers, some of you might be interested in comparing it with the linear regression model. Let's assume that you have a group of women with a breast lump who are to receive a biopsy when the lump will then be diagnosed as malignant or benign. We will let this binary diagnosis be our *outcome variable* Y, so $Y = 0$ (benign) or $Y = 1$ (malignant). We will have two explanatory variables (although there could be more), $X_1 = $ age and $X_2 = $ whether has ever smoked. The logistic regression equation is written:

$$P(Y = 1) = e^{(\beta_0 + \beta_1 X_1 + \beta_2 X_2 + \ldots)} \bigg/ \left[1 + e^{(\beta_0 + \beta_1 X_1 + \beta_2 X_2 + \ldots)} \right]$$

Where $P(Y = 1)$ is the probability that $Y = 1$, i.e. the probability of a malignant diagnosis. As with linear regression, the independent variables can be any mixture of metric, ordinal or nominal. e is the exponent operator (you will have an e^x button on your calculator). Notice that the term in brackets is just the same as in the linear regression model. The βs are the population regression parameters, as before.

We can't use the linear regression model with a binary outcome variable because there is no guarantee that Y will only take the values between 0 and 1 as required for a probability value. The above logistic equation does the trick.

VARIABLE SELECTION AND MODEL ESTIMATION

The model building situation is much the same as with the linear regression model (see previous chapter). Either the researcher has little idea which explanatory variables might be relevant so the list of candidate variables is long. Or a particular hypothesis is to be tested, i.e. the explanatory variable of principal focus is already identified and potential confounders are known from the literature.

Variable selection procedures are also similar to those used with linear regression (see the relevant section in Chapter 24). That is, either forward, backwards, stepwise methods for automated estimation, with the limitations previously noted, but which maybe more appropriate if little is known about which

Understanding Clinical Papers Second Edition   David Bowers, Allan House, David Owens
© 2006 John Wiley & Sons, Ltd

variables might be relevant. Or manual selection, which as we have seen offers more control of the model building process, helps with the identification of potential confounders, and is appropriate if a particular hypothesis is to be examined. There is, however, one change in the criteria used to include/exclude variables. In linear regression we included variables with a p-value <0.05, and excluded them otherwise unless their removal changes any coefficient value by some noticeable amount. In logistic regression we may be more interested in the change in the odds ratio (see below). As an example of the above, Figure 25.1 is an extract from a clinical paper on eczema and endotoxin exposure in infants. The outcome variable was 'Has eczema (yes or no)'.

INTERPRETATION AND STATISTICAL SIGNIFICANCE OF THE REGRESSION COEFFICIENTS

In the linear regression model we use p-values and confidence intervals (based on the t-test) to determine whether the regression coefficients (β_1, β_2, etc.) are statistically significant. The value of these coefficients are also of interest because they tell us by how much the outcome variable will change for each unit change in the associated explanatory variable.

In the logistic regression model researchers can use the p-value of the *Wald* test (related to the chi-squared distribution) to tell us whether the estimated coefficients are statistically significant or not. However, we are not now as interested in the *value* of the coefficients, as we are in the value of the corresponding odds ratio (OR), and *its* statistical significance (p-value <0.05, or confidence interval not including 1). In logistic regression a change of one unit in an independent variable causes a change of β in the log of the odds ratio – so not easy to interpret. However, if we raise e to the power of β, we get the odds ratio! That is, $OR = e^{\beta}$. This is usually provided for us in the results, hopefully with the corresponding confidence interval.

To illustrate these ideas, Figure 25.2 is from a study of the risk factors for depression symptoms in long-term care residents in Taiwan. The outcome variable was, 'Has depressive symptoms (yes or no)'.

As you can see, only three risk factors turned out to be statistically significant, Type of institution ($OR = 1.678$), Functional status ($OR = 0.987$), and Impaired swallowing ($OR = 1.686$). So a resident with impaired swallowing has nearly 1.7 the odds of having depressive symptoms than a resident

Endotoxin Exposure and Eczema in the First Year of Life

Phipatanakul W, Celedon JC, Raby BA, Litonjua AA, Milton DK, Sredl D, Weiss ST and Gold DR

Logistic regression was used to study the relationship between predictor variables and eczema in the first year of life while controlling for potential confounders and examining interactions. Stepwise logistic regression was used to develop the multivariate models. In the final models we included those variables that satisfied a change-in-estimate criterion ($\leq 10\%$ in the odds ratio) or that were significant at the P < 0.05 level.

The authors in this study of eczema and endotoxin exposure, used the stepwise estimation method to select the variables in their logistic model.

FIGURE 25.1   Variable selection methods in a study of eczema and endotoxin exposure in 1st year of life

Depressive symptoms in long-term care residents in Taiwan

Li-Chan Lin, Tyng-Guey Wang, Miao-Yen Chen, Shiao-Chi Wu and Portwood MJ

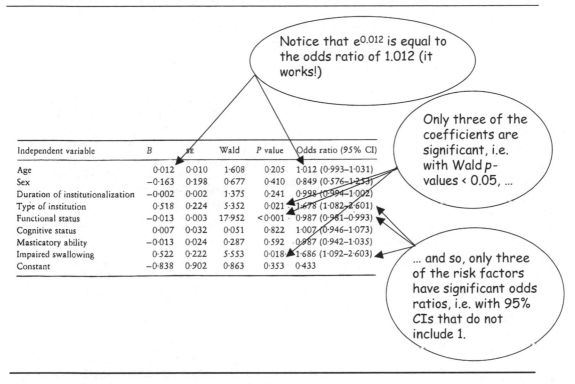

FIGURE 25.2   Results of logistic regression analysis of risk factors for depression in long-term care residents in Taiwan

without impaired swallowing. Notice that the logistic regression coefficient for the risk factor 'impaired swallowing' has a value of 0.522.

If we raise e to the power 0.522, i.e., $e^{0.522}$, the result is 1.686 – which is equal to the odds ratio for this risk factor. A similar result can be demonstrated for all the other regression coefficients and their respective odds ratios.

DUMMY VARIABLES

The treatment of nominal variables also mirrors that with the linear regression model. Nominal variables must be coded, but ordinal and metric variables can be entered 'as is' (unless there are questions about the linearity of a relationship – see previous chapter). Authors should provide information about any coding used, and identify the reference category.

As an example of the use of dummy variables in logistic regression, Figure 25.3 is from a study into overweight children and iron deficiency. The outcome variable was 'Iron deficient (yes or no)', and the model had six independent variables: two metric (age, and BMI percentile), two ordinal (poverty status, and educational level of carer), and two nominal (gender, and race/ethnicity).

Overweight Children and Adolescents: A Risk Group for Iron Deficiency

Nead Karen G, Halterman Jill S, Kaczorowski Jeoffrey M, Auinger Peggy, and Weitzman Michael

	Odds Ratio	95% CI	P Value
Age			
2–5 y	1.2	0.7–2.2	.4
6–11 y	1.0		
12–16 y	2.6	1.4–4.6	.002
Gender			
Female	2.6	1.7–3.9	< .0001
Male	1.0		
Race/ethnicity			
White	1.0		
Black	1.3	0.7–2.2	.3
Mexican American	3.5	2.2–5.8	< 0.0001
Other	3.8	2.0–7.1	< 0.0001
Poverty status			
Below poverty line	2.0	0.9–4.2	.06
Above poverty line	1.0		
Care-taker education			
< 12th grade	0.7	0.3–1.5	.4
12th grade	1.0	0.5–2.0	.9
> 12th grade	1.0		
BMI percentile			
< 85%	1.0		
≥ 85% to < 95%	2.0	1.2–3.5	.01
≥ 95%	2.3	1.4–3.9	0.002

The authors have used dummy variables for all six risk factors, including age and BMI, which are metric, and education of care-taker (ordinal), perhaps because they suspected a non-linear relationship with iron deficiency.

We know White is the reference category here because it has an OR=1, and no CI or p-value is given.

A child with a BMI in the ≥ 95% percentile has 2.3 times the odds of being iron deficient than a child in the reference category - the < 85% BMI percentile. This OR is significant because the 95% CI does not contain 1.

FIGURE 25.3   Results from a logistic regression of iron deficiency in overweight children. The outcome variable is 'Iron deficiency Yes/No'. There are six explanatory variables, all of which have been expressed as dummies

In Figure 25.3 the authors have chosen to categorize and code as dummy variables: age (three categories – reference category is the middle category); care-taker education (three categories – reference is third category); and BMI percentile (three categories – reference is first category). Each of these variables will have been represented in the model with two dummy variables, one less than the number of categories. The authors do not give reasons for this categorizing, presumably because they knew or suspected non-linear relationships with the outcome variable. Finally race/ethnicity is nominal so *has* to be represented by dummy variables (three dummies for the four categories). Gender (nominal) and poverty status (ordinal) each have only two categories so will be represented by a single dummy (0/1) variable.

The results in Figure 25.3 show that Age is not a risk factor for iron deficiency in 2–5 year olds, the confidence interval includes 1, but is a statistically significant risk factor for children aged 12–16. These have 2.6 times the odds of iron deficiency as the 6–11-year-olds – the reference class (confidence interval does not include 1). Gender is a statistically significant risk factor, girls have 2.6 times the odds of iron deficiency as boys – the reference class (confidence interval does not include 1).

GOODNESS OF FIT

We saw that in the linear regression model the goodness of fit of the model is measured by R^2. In the logistic regression model goodness of fit is most commonly measured either by the Pearson chi-squared statistic, χ^2, or by the Hosmer-Lemeshow statistic, C, (Hosmer and Lemeshow, 1989), both of which can be tested using the p-value associated with the chi-squared test (although neither measure is commonly quoted). The null hypothesis is that the model *is* the correct fit. As an example, the following is an extract from a study of severe malnutrition among hospitalised children in rural Kenya: 'We evaluated the performance of the resulting models using the Hosmer-Lemeshow goodness-of-fit test,' and they later report that the 'Hosmer-Lemeshow goodness-of-fit test $\chi^2 = 8.90$, p = 0.18.' Thus the hypothesis of a good fit is not rejected.

EFFECT MODIFICATION – INTERACTION

The same warnings apply here as in the linear regression model (see Chapter 24). Interaction terms adversely affect parsimony (particularly with dummy variables) and may lead to problems associated with sample size. Only if they have *strong* clinical justification should authors include interaction terms in their model.

MODEL DIAGNOSTICS

In linear regression not only do we want authors to report a measure of the goodness of fit of their model to the data (R^2), we also hope that they will demonstrate the linearity of the relationship, and in addition show that they have examined the shape of the error term (Normal with constant variance), as a check on some of the basic assumptions of the model, sometimes called *model diagnostics*. As we noted though, this doesn't often happen.

In logistic regression, model diagnostics are much more complex. Because of the binary nature of the outcome variable, the error term is not Normally distributed (it does, in fact, have a binomial distribution – which we haven't touched on). Nor is its variance constant over the range of each independent variable, but on the contrary it is *related* to their probability distributions. See how difficult it soon gets! In addition, the logistic model does not have the set of necessary conditions seen in linear regression, apart from the obvious – that the outcome variable has to be binary (self-evident). There are model diagnostic procedures available, a lot of them graphical in nature, which are largely concerned with the data patterns in the explanatory variables and the consequences of deleting one or more of these patterns on goodness of fit and so on. Because of these problems, it is extremely rare to see any logistic model diagnostics in clinical papers. If you want to know more about the possibilities, try Hosmer and Lemeshow (1989), or Field (2000).

26

Systematic Review and Meta-analysis

If you were dealing with a patient with a particular condition and you wanted to find out the current consensus on the most appropriate treatment, you might look through all the relevant journals that you could get your hands on, and identify those studies that deal with treatment for this condition. If you had easy access to one or more clinical database – such as Medline, Embase, or CINAHL (Cumulative Index to Nursing & Allied Health Literature) – your job would be that much easier. Because your interest is in treatments, it would make sense to concentrate on the findings from well-conducted clinical trials (Chapter 6) because they generally offer the best protection against confounding bias (Chapter 10). Unfortunately, three problems are very likely to arise (unless of course there have been no trials of treatment in this area):

- Many of the studies that you discover will be based on participants who are highly selected and probably unrepresentative of typical patients – so it may be tricky to generalize the findings to your practice.
- Many of the studies that you discover will be based on smallish samples which, as we have seen earlier, leads to imprecise and unreliable findings.
- Partly as a consequence of the above problems, many of the trials come to differing and conflicting conclusions.

One possible response to these three difficulties is to identify all relevant trials and then combine them into one big study with a single overall finding which, drawn as it is from a much larger sample, is thereby more precise. The final bottom line will usually be made up of many studies and so gets closer to representing the real-world population of patients – because the highly selected patient groups in one trial are quite unlike the highly selected patients in another; a wide range of study populations have been sampled by a wide range of researchers.

In practice, clinicians do not usually do any of the above, relying instead on others to undertake the work. Increasingly, the world of health care is compiling and disseminating reviews of effectiveness across the whole array of treatments. These reviews often incorporate critical appraisal of the quality of the trials and sometimes go as far as to make recommendations to health-care staff – at times even guidelines that carry the seal of approval of health departments or others who fund the patients' care. This book does not tackle this literature, often deemed part of *evidence-based practice*: there are many books and websites available that do. But we do regard the explanation of these *systematic reviews* of trials as an important part of our guide to understanding clinical papers, and the rest of this chapter is a guide to some of the procedures used by systematic reviewers. In particular, we deal with the numerical amalgamation of individual trials, known as *meta-analysis*.

SYSTEMATIC REVIEW

A written review of treatments for a condition can amount to the opinion of its authors, backed up by findings that support that opinion. Of course, where the author is an acknowledged expert, the message

Understanding Clinical Papers Second Edition David Bowers, Allan House, David Owens
© 2006 John Wiley & Sons, Ltd

emerging from the review might be supported by his or her own research together with that of his or her chums; research from the wider world might be cited when it agrees with the author's view but ignored when it does not. Plainly, such a review would not be a satisfactory guide to treatment. Instead, it would be better were the review to have followed a strict protocol that sets out how the reviewer ensured that as much of the relevant literature as possible has been searched and that the applicable findings are all appraised for quality before synthesis into the final version. In short, this kind of systematic review mimics a primary research study: it has a specific question to answer and its methods are made clear (including the steps taken to minimize bias), such that the work could be replicated by another reviewer.

In the extract from a systematic review shown as an example here (Figure 26.1) there is a clearly stated question. The primary research studies that were to be included are described in a few words but with great clarity: they have to have a certain kind of design; certain standards for the allocation of the treatments have to be met; the intervention has to be of a narrowly-defined type; and benefit has to be measured in a certain way. There are also some sensible and explicit exclusions. The reader is told how

Systematic review of dietary intervention trials to lower blood total cholesterol in free-living subjects

J L Tang, J M Armitage, T Lancaster, C A Silagy, G H Fowler, H A W Neil

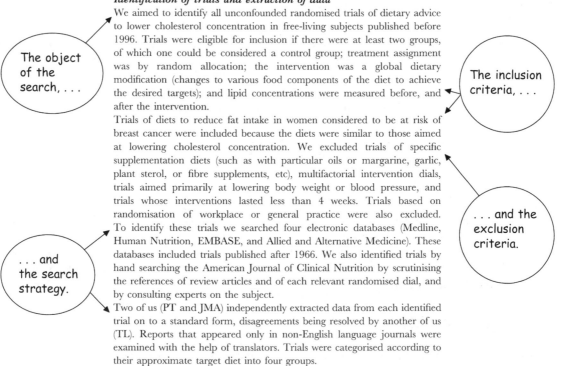

Methods

Identification of trials and extraction of data

We aimed to identify all unconfounded randomised trials of dietary advice to lower cholesterol concentration in free-living subjects published before 1996. Trials were eligible for inclusion if there were at least two groups, of which one could be considered a control group; treatment assignment was by random allocation; the intervention was a global dietary modification (changes to various food components of the diet to achieve the desired targets); and lipid concentrations were measured before, and after the intervention.

Trials of diets to reduce fat intake in women considered to be at risk of breast cancer were included because the diets were similar to those aimed at lowering cholesterol concentration. We excluded trials of specific supplementation diets (such as with particular oils or margarine, garlic, plant sterol, or fibre supplements, etc), multifactorial intervention dials, trials aimed primarily at lowering body weight or blood pressure, and trials whose interventions lasted less than 4 weeks. Trials based on randomisation of workplace or general practice were also excluded. To identify these trials we searched four electronic databases (Medline, Human Nutrition, EMBASE, and Allied and Alternative Medicine). These databases included trials published after 1966. We also identified trials by hand searching the American Journal of Clinical Nutrition by scrutinising the references of review articles and of each relevant randomised dial, and by consulting experts on the subject.

Two of us (PT and JMA) independently extracted data from each identified trial on to a standard form, disagreements being resolved by another of us (TL). Reports that appeared only in non-English language journals were examined with the help of translators. Trials were categorised according to their approximate target diet into four groups.

Text in circles: The object of the search, ... | ... and the search strategy. | The inclusion criteria, ... | ... and the exclusion criteria.

FIGURE 26.1   Authors' description of their search strategy and the inclusion and exclusion criteria in a study into dietary intervention and blood cholesterol

the authors searched the biomedical literature (and the literature on alternative health treatments) and something about how the findings are extracted.

Figure 26.1 does not state that the quality of the studies was appraised by the authors. Figure 26.2 on the other hand, shows part of the Abstract for a systematic review that does refer to this process of appraising methodological quality. The main text (not shown) describes in more detail how the reviewers used three criteria to judge the quality (concealment of allocation, blinding of outcome assessment, and handling of withdrawals and dropouts) – together with the overall quality of reporting and handling of data in the trials. You might notice that these three criteria are ones that we have paid attention to earlier in this book, when dealing with trials (in Chapter 6).

Local treatments for cutaneous warts

Gibbs, S; Harvey, I; Sterling, JC; Stark, R
Cochrane Database of Systematic Reviews

Background:
Viral warts caused by the human papilloma virus represent one of the most common diseases of the skin. Any area of skin can be affected although the hands and feet are by far the commonest sites. A very wide range of local treatments are available.

Objectives:
To assess the effects of different local treatments for cutaneous, non-genital warts in healthy people.

Search strategy:
We searched the Cochrane Controlled Trials Register (January 2003), the Skin Group trials register (January 2003), MEDLINE (1966 to January 2003), EMBASE (1980 to January 2003) and a number of other key biomedical and health economics databases. In addition the cited references of all trials identified and key review articles were searched. Pharmaceutical companies involved in local treatments for warts and experts in the field were contacted. The most recent searches were carried

Selection criteria:
Randomised controlled trials of local treatments for cutaneous non-genital viral warts in immunocompetent human hosts were included.

Data collection and analysis:
Study selection and assessment of methodological quality were carried out by two independent reviewers.

Main results:
Fifty-two trials were identified which fulfilled the criteria for inclusion in the review. The evidence provided by these studies was generally weak because of poor methodology and reporting. In 17 trials with placebo groups that used participants as the unit of analysis the average cure rate of placebo preparations was 30% (range 0 to 73%) after an average period of 10 weeks (range 4 to 24 weeks). . . . . .

The Cochrane Library contains thousands of systematic reviews and has information about hundreds of thousands of randomized trials

In this review, the reviewers assessed the quality of each trial that was included. The main text of the review gives details of how they did it.

FIGURE 26.2   A Cochrane Review of local treatments for skin warts, showing that the included studies were assessed for their quality

The example in Figure 26.2 is taken from the Cochrane Library, which is an electronic database that is largely dedicated to the publication of systematic reviews. It is a tremendously rich source of reviewed and appraised evidence about health-care interventions of all kinds, and it sets very high standards for the reviews that it publishes. It also contains many useful sources of guidance concerning searching, reviewing, combining and appraising research.

PUBLICATION AND OTHER BIASES

The success of any systematic review depends critically on how thorough and wide-ranging the search for relevant studies is. One frequently quoted difficulty is that of *publication bias*, which can arise from a number of sources:

- There is a tendency for journals to favour the acceptance of studies showing positive outcomes at the expense of those with negative outcomes.
- There is a tendency for authors to favour the submission to journals of studies showing positive outcomes at the expense of those with negative outcomes.
- Studies with positive results are more likely to be published in English language journals, giving them a better chance of capture in the search process.
- Studies with positive results are more likely to be cited, giving them a better chance of capture in the search process.
- Studies with positive results are more likely to be published in more than one journal, giving them a better chance of capture in the search process.
- Some studies are never submitted for publication, for example, those which fail to show a positive result, those by pharmaceutical companies (particularly if the results are unfavourable), graduate dissertations, and so on.

There are a number of other sources of potential bias. *Inclusion bias*, for example, arises from the possibility that inclusion and exclusion criteria will be set to favour the admission of studies with particular outcomes over less 'helpful' studies. A further potential problem is that smaller studies tend to be less methodologically sound, with wider variability in outcomes, and are consequently less reliable. Moreover, lower-quality studies tend to show larger effects. In the light of all this, it is important that the paper should contain clear evidence that the authors have addressed these issues. One possibility is for them to provide a *funnel plot*.

THE FUNNEL PLOT

In a funnel plot the size of the study is represented on the vertical axis and the size of the treatment's effect (in this case represented by the odds ratio) on the horizontal axis. In the absence of bias, the funnel plot should have the shape of a *symmetric* upturned funnel. Larger studies shown at the top of the funnel will be more precise (their results will not be so spread out), smaller studies, shown towards the bottom, less precise, and therefore more spread out. These differences produce the funnel shape. However, if the funnel is asymmetrical – for example, if parts of the funnel are missing or poorly represented – then this is suggestive of bias of one form or another.

A large clinical trial tends to be published whatever it finds because lots of people and a lot of money will have been needed to carry it out, so its very existence will be known to many; failure to publish a large trial because the results disappoint some of those involved will lead to adverse scrutiny and comment. Small studies, on the other hand, are often not published, and few people know (or care) about the consequent loss to the literature. Publication bias therefore arises especially with smaller studies and, as described above, would usually be expected to lead to the preferential publication of trials showing effects that favour active or new treatments (rather than placebos or treatment-as-usual). The clever characteristic of the funnel plot is that its design locates the missing blobs – due to publication bias – down near the base of the funnel (where the small studies are plotted) and towards the side that represents benefit for the placebo or treatment-as-usual.

For example, in the following study, the authors were reporting the results of a meta-analysis into the use of β-blockers as a secondary prevention after myocardial infarction. The resulting funnel plot is shown in Figure 26.3.

Each point in Figure 26.3 represents one of the studies. Values to the left of the value 1 on the horizontal axis show reductions in mortality, values to the right show increases. The congregation of values around 0.78 (about 80%) indicates an overall 20% reduction in the odds of mortality. The authors comment as follows:

> The funnel plot is shown in [Figure 26.3]. Visual assessment shows some asymmetry, which indicates that there was selective non-publication of smaller trials with less sizeable benefit. However, in formal statistical analysis the degree of asymmetry is found to be small and non-significant (P > 0.1). Furthermore, exclusion of the smaller studies had little effect on the overall estimate. Bias does not therefore seem to have distorted the findings from this meta-analysis.

Bias in location and selection of studies

Mathias Egger, George Davey Smith

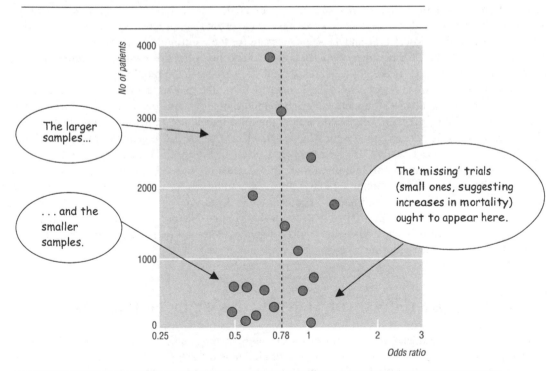

FIGURE 26.3   Funnel plot used to check for publication bias, in a meta-analysis of β-blockers to prevent secondary myocardial infarction

HETEROGENEITY

Even when a set of potentially similar studies has been identified, authors have to make sure they are similar enough to be combined. For example, they should have similar subjects, have the same type and level of intervention, the same output measure, the same treatment effect, and so on. The underlying assumption (i.e. the null hypothesis) of meta-analysis is that all the studies measure the same effect in the same population, and that any difference between them is due to chance alone. When the results are combined, the chance element cancels out. Only if studies are *homogenous* in this way can they be properly combined.

You might find the comments on heterogeneity by the authors of the diet and cholesterol study quoted earlier illuminating:

> The design and results of these dietary studies differed greatly. They were conducted over 30 years and varied in their aims, in the intensity and type of intervention, and in the different baseline characteristics of the subjects included. Completeness and duration of follow up also differed. Unsurprisingly, the heterogeneity between their effects on blood cholesterol concentration was also significant. Among the longer trials some, but not all, of the heterogeneity between the effects on blood cholesterol concentration seemed to be due to the type of diet recommended. Deciding which trials should be included in which groups is open to different interpretation and, although we tried to be consistent, for some trials the target diets either were not clearly stated or did not fit neatly into recognised categories such as the step 1 and 2 diets. It is important to be cautious in interpreting meta-analysis when there is evidence of significant heterogeneity; although there was no evidence that the overall results were influenced by trials with outlying values   (Tang *et al.* 1998)

Authors should present some evidence that the homogeneity assumption has been tested. One possibility is for them to provide readers with a *L'Abbé plot* (see Figure 26.4). The L'Abbé plot displays *outcomes* from a number of studies, with the percentage of successes (or the event rate, or reduction in risk, etc.) with the treatment group on the vertical axis, and the same measure for the control/placebo group on the horizontal axis. The 45° line is thus the boundary between effective and non-effective treatment. Values above the line show beneficial results. If possible, authors should use varying sized plotting points proportional to sample size (not done in this example). The compactness of the plot is a measure of the degree of heterogeneity across the studies; the more compact, the more homogenous the studies. The *overall* meta-analytic result can also of course be plotted on the same plot (but is not shown in Figure 26.4).

A more commonly used alternative is the *Mantel–Haenszel test for heterogeneity*, which uses the chi-squared distribution (see Chapter 21). An example is given in Figure 26.5, taken from a study which 'aimed to identify and evaluate all published randomised trials of hospital versus general practice care for people with diabetes'. The author's Table 2 presents a summary of the weighted (by sample size) mean differences for a number of different outcomes. Table 3 presents similar information for different outcomes in terms of the odds ratio. The *p*-values for the Mantel–Haenszel test (using chi-squared) are given in the last column. Only one set of studies displays evidence of heterogeneity, but since this comprised only two studies, the result is somewhat meaningless.

COMBINING THE STUDIES: THE MANTEL–HAENSZEL PROCEDURE

The final step if a meta-analysis is required is to *combine* the studies using the Mantel–Haenszel procedure (which we do not describe) to produce a single-value overall summary of the net effect across all studies, as in the next example (note that this is not to be confused with the Mantel–Haenszel test for heterogeneity). In Figure 26.6 the authors were reporting a meta-analysis of randomized controlled trials to compare antibiotic with placebo for acute cough in adults. They focused on placebo-controlled trials

Quantitive systematic review of topically applied non-steroidal anti-inflammatory drugs

R A Moore, M R Tramèr, D Carroll, P J Wiffen, H J McQuay

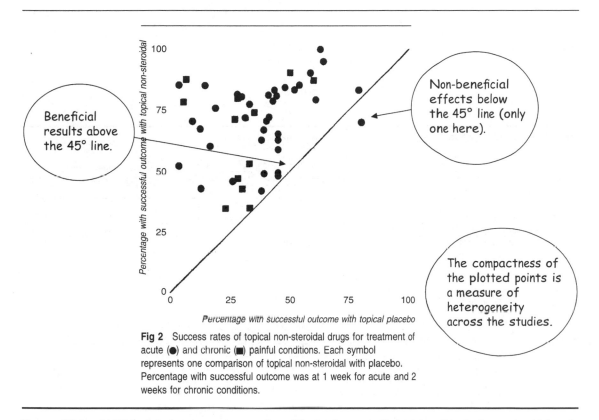

Fig 2 Success rates of topical non-steroidal drugs for treatment of acute (●) and chronic (■) painful conditions. Each symbol represents one comparison of topical non-steroidal with placebo. Percentage with successful outcome was at 1 week for acute and 2 weeks for chronic conditions.

FIGURE 26.4 L'Abbé plot showing outcomes from 37 placebo-controlled trials of topical non-steroidal anti-inflammatory drugs in acute and chronic pain conditions

that reported three specific outcomes: the proportion of subjects reporting productive cough; the proportion of subjects reporting no improvement at follow-up; and the proportion of subjects with side-effects.

The authors' *forest plots* for the first two of these outcomes showing the risk ratios (called by the authors 'relative risks') in favour of the specific outcome are shown in Figure 26.6. The forest plot (sometimes referred to irreverently as a 'blobbogram') is a graph of study outcome on the vertical axis (often arranged in order of effect) versus outcome measure on the horizontal axis. The outcome measure might be odds or risk ratios, means or proportions or their differences, event rates, and so on. Each study is often represented by a box with a horizontal line through it, which represents the width of the 95% confidence interval. The area of each box should be proportional to its sample size.

The overall net outcome effect is shown with a diamond shape by these authors (one for each of the two outcomes). The area of the diamond is proportional to the total number of studies represented, and the width the 95% confidence interval. Values to the left of an odds ratio of 1 (bottom axis) show

Diabetes care in general practice: meta-analysis of randomised control trials

Simon Griffin

P-values for tests of heterogeneity across studies for a number of different outcomes.

Table 2 Summary weighted differences comparing prompted general practice care with hospital care

Outcome	Weighted difference in mean values (95% CI)		χ^2 test of between trial heterogeneity	P value
	Favours prompted GP care	Favours hospital care		
Glycated haemoglobin (%) (3 trials, n=535)	−0.28 (−0.59 to 0.03)		3.90	>0.10
Systolic blood pressure (mm Hg) (2 trials, n=369)		1.62 (−3.30 to 6.53)	2.56	>0.10
Diastolic blood pressure (mm Hg) (2 trials, n=369)		0.56 (−1.69 to 2.80)	0.10	>0.75
Frequency of review (per patient per year) (2 trials, n=402)	0.27 (0.07 to 0.47)		0.59	>0.30
Frequency of glycated haemoglobin test (per patient per year) (2 trials, n=402)	1.60 (1.45 to 1.75)		0.05	>0.80

Table 3 Summary odds ratios comparing prompted general practice care with hospital care

Outcome	Odds ratios (95% CI)		χ^2 test of between trial heterogeneity	P value
	Favours prompted GP care	Favours hospital care		
Mortality (2 trials, n=456)		1.06 (0.53 to 2.11)	0.0	1.0
Losses to follow up (3 trials, n=589)	0.37 (0.22 to 0.61)		1.63	>0.30
Referral to chiropody (2 trials, n=399)	2.51 (1.59 to 3.97)		9.77	<0.005
Referral to dietitian (2 trials, n=399)		0.61 (0.40 to 0.92)	0.56	>0.30

The only heterogeneity is across the chiropody studies (but there are only two of these!).

FIGURE 26.5 The Mantel–Haenszel test for heterogeneity in studies with differing outcomes in the diabetes care study. The null hypothesis is that the studies are homogenous. Only one outcome (chiropody) has significant heterogeneity

reductions in fatalities among cases, those to the right an increase in fatalities (compared with control groups).

The Mantel–Haenszel procedure was used to produce the final result shown at the bottom of the forest plot in Figure 26.6. The aggregate relative risks are 0.85 for productive cough and 0.62 for no improvement at follow-up, reductions in the risk for each of these conditions which appear to favour the antibiotic over the placebo. However, since both have 95% confidence intervals which include 1, neither is in fact significant, confirmed by the fact that both diamonds cross the line where relative risk = 1. In

Quantitative systematic review of randomised controlled trials comparing antibiotic with placebo for acute cough in adults

Tom Fahey, Nigel Stocks, Toby Thomas

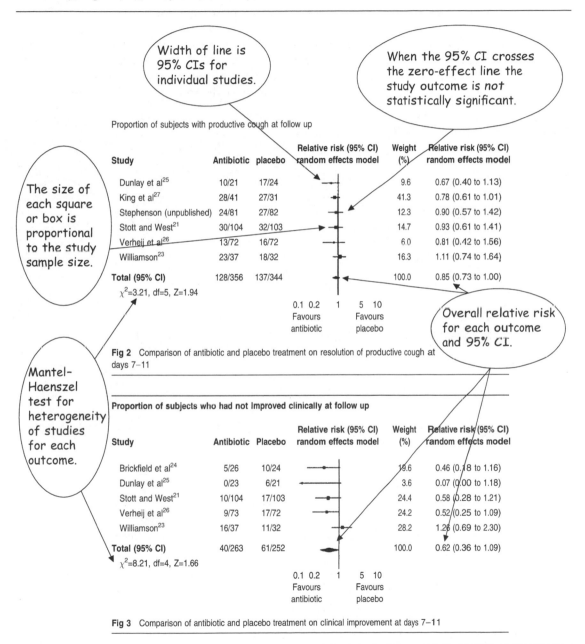

Fig 2 Comparison of antibiotic and placebo treatment on resolution of productive cough at days 7–11

Fig 3 Comparison of antibiotic and placebo treatment on clinical improvement at days 7–11

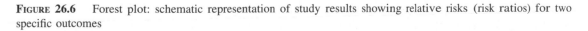

FIGURE 26.6 Forest plot: schematic representation of study results showing relative risks (risk ratios) for two specific outcomes

other words, the efficacy of antibiotic over placebo for acute cough in this population is not established by this meta-analysis.

Notice that heterogeneity test results are also provided, but unfortunately the authors have chosen to give us neither confidence intervals nor p-values for these tests. Instead they report the value of what is called the *z-statistic*. However, this is easily interpreted. The rule of thumb is that z should be greater than 2.2 for the null hypothesis to be rejected, i.e. for us to reject the assumption of homogeneity across the studies. In this case, since both z values are less than 2, it is reasonably safe to assume that the studies for both outcomes are homogenous.

The number of meta-analytic studies in the journals has increased steadily over the past few years. With the increasing favour of evidence-based practice, this trend is likely to accelerate. However, not all researchers are unreservedly enthusiastic about this procedure, and worry about various shortcomings (due to bias and other problems). Unfortunately we do not have the space to devote to these ideas.

27

Measuring Survival

Clinicians are often interested in questions relating to the survival time of patients following some clinical episode. For example, what is the probability that a patient diagnosed with lung cancer will survive for 12 months? Or which alternative treatments will offer a patient a longer survival time? These are the sorts of questions at which *survival analysis* is aimed. In essence, a sample of patients is regularly monitored from the time of some clinical event for some given period of time or until the study finishes. The time taken by each patient to reach some defined clinical outcome or end-point is recorded. An *end-point* might be death, or relapse, or repeat of episode, or recovery, and so on.

Of course, it is quite possible that some patients may not reach the end-point before the end of the study period. For example, if the end-point is death within one year, we might find that 20% of the subjects are still alive at this time. The problem is that we don't know how long these subjects will go on living nor therefore their true survival time. The data on subjects such as these are said to be *censored*. Censoring can also occur if subjects withdraw from the study before it is completed, for example, they may relocate, or die from a non-related cause. A second difficulty is that subjects may not all enter the study at the same time and some of the more recent recruits may be observed for a shorter time period. The problem of censored observations, compounded by unequal observation periods, makes the analysis of such data somewhat tricky. We can't, for example, calculate the mean survival time, since we don't know all the survival times. We can, however, estimate the median survival time, as you will see shortly.

In this chapter we will discuss ways in which these and other problems may be overcome, and at the same time explain some of the ideas and terms which you may encounter in clinical papers reporting the results of survival studies. We start with a commonly used procedure for describing the survival experience of one or more groups of patients, the Kaplan–Meier method.

THE KAPLAN–MEIER METHOD – MEDIAN SURVIVAL TIME

The basis of the Kaplan–Meier method is a *life table* which contains the chronological progress of the subjects in the study, noting how many experience the end-point of interest every day (or week, month, etc.), how many withdraw prematurely, and what proportion remain. The information in the table is often presented by authors in the form of the Kaplan–Meier curve (which actually looks more like a staircase).

The method enables researchers (i) to calculate the survival time for any given proportion of the sample, along with a confidence interval for the survival proportion; (ii) to calculate the probability of survival; or (iii) to compare the difference in the proportions surviving in two or more groups (along with the appropriate confidence interval).

An example of the Kaplan–Meier procedure is shown in Figure 27.1, and is from a study into the survival of children with high-grade malignant gliomas and their expression of the p53 protein.

In their paper the authors state that the prognosis of children with high-grade gliomas is uncertain, but expressed the belief that the degree of expression of the p53 protein might be associated with progression-free survival. They followed the progress of children, grouped as having an over-expression of p53 or not, and plotted Kaplan–Meier curves for the end-point of *progression-free survival* over time, for both groups.

Understanding Clinical Papers Second Edition   David Bowers, Allan House, David Owens
© 2006 John Wiley & Sons, Ltd

EXPRESSION OF p53 AND PROGNOSIS IN CHILDREN WITH MALIGNANT GLIOMAS

Pollack IF, Finkelstein SD, Woods J, Burnham J, Holmes EJ, Hamilton RL, Yates AJ, Boyett JM, Finlay JL and Sposto R

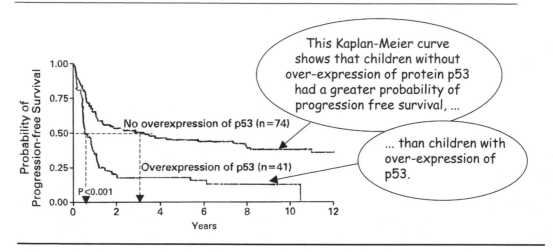

FIGURE 27.1   Kaplan–Meier curves showing the probability of progression-free survival in two groups of children with malignant glioma, one group showing over-expression of protein p53 (bottom curve), the other not (top curve)

As you can see, the probability of progression-free survival was noticeably higher in the group of children without the over-expression of p53 (top curve). Notice that the Kaplan–Meier curve is of a step form (not particularly easy to see in these two curves), this reflects the discrete nature of the end-point. The *median* probability values for progression-free survival are found on the time axis corresponding to where the horizontal 0.5 (50%) line cuts the two curves. This gives median probabilities corresponding to about 6 months (over-expression of p53) and three years (no over-expression of the protein).

COMPARING SURVIVAL IN TWO GROUPS

Perhaps the most frequent application of survival analysis reported in clinical papers is the comparison of two groups. In the following study (Figure 27.2) the authors compared the survival experience of two groups of women diagnosed between 1981 and 1986 with breast cancer. One group had bone-marrow micrometastases evident at diagnosis, the other group had not. The hypothesis was that the presence of bone-marrow micrometastases reduced the chances of survival.

The authors report that by the end of 1995, of the 89 patients with micrometastases 57 (64%) had died, and of the 261 patients without micrometastases 122 (47%) had died. The *p*-value for this percentage difference in survival was 0.001, which is of course statistically significant. Survival from breast cancer seems better among those with no evidence of micrometastases.

THE LOG-RANK TEST

In the study quoted above, the authors compared the proportions surviving in the two groups by presenting a Kaplan–Meier curve for each group, and calculating a confidence interval for the difference in the proportions surviving at the end of 1995. The shortcoming of this approach is that it compares survival at some *arbitrary* point in time.

Outcome of primary-breast-cancer patients with micrometastases: a long-term follow-up study

Janine L Mansi, Helen Gogas, Judith M Bliss, Jean-Claude Gazet, Uta Berger, R Charles Coombes

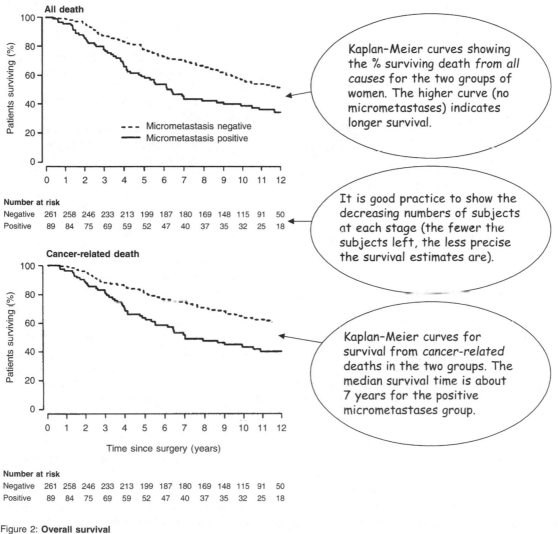

Figure 2: **Overall survival**

FIGURE 27.2 Kaplan–Meier curves for the overall survival of patients diagnosed with breast cancer, with and without micrometastases at original presentation. Notice that the median survival time from cancer-related death cannot be determined for the 'no micrometastases' group (top curve in bottom figure) because this curve does not reach the 50% surviving value on the vertical axis

Efficacy of azithromycin in prevention of *Pneumocystis carinii* pneumonia: a randomised trial

Michael W Dunne, Samuel Bozzette, J Allen McCutchan, Michael P Dubé, Fred R Sattler, Donald Forthal Carol A Kemper, Diane Havlir, for the California Collaborative Treatment Group

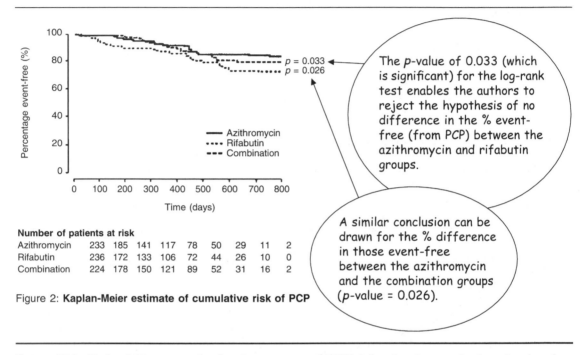

Figure 2: **Kaplan-Meier estimate of cumulative risk of PCP**

FIGURE 27.3 Kaplan–Meier curves showing the percentage of HIV-1 infected patients randomly assigned to three groups (the first group given azithromycin, the second rifabutin, and the third a combination of both drugs), who were event-free (from *Pneumocystitis carinii* pneumonia or PCP). *p*-values are for the log-rank test of no difference in the percentage event-free (no PCP) between the azithromycin group on the one hand, and the rifabutin and combination groups respectively

To discriminate between the *complete survival experience* of two (or more) groups, the *log-rank test*, which uses the chi-squared distribution, is more appropriate. The hypothesis to be tested is that the different groups are in fact from the same population; that is, have the same survival experience.

In the following study (see Figure 27.3) the authors were concerned to assess the clinical efficacy of azithromycin for prophylaxis of *Pneumocystis carinii* pneumonia in HIV-1 infected patients. Patients were randomly assigned to one of three treatment groups: the first group given azithromycin, the second rifabutin, and the third a combination of both drugs. The authors present Kaplan–Meier curves for the three treatment groups showing the event-free (no *P. carinii* pneumonia) survival experiences over an 800-day period.

They used the log-rank test to test the hypothesis that there is no difference in the percentage event-free between the azithromycin and rifabutin groups (*p*-value = 0.033), and between the azithromycin and the combination groups (*p*-value = 0.026). The authors concluded that azithromycin as prophylaxis for *P. carinii* pneumonia provides additional protection over and above standard *P. carinii* pneumonia prophylaxis. However, these results should be treated with caution because of the very small size of the survivor group towards the end of the study.

Incidentally, the p-value for the log-rank test is also shown in Figure 27.1 as, 'P < 0.001', indicating a statistically significant difference in the survival times of the two groups of children with glioma with and without over-expression of p. 53.

LOG-RANK TEST FOR TREND

The only difference between the three groups in the example in Figure 27.3 was their drug treatment. However, some groups will be ordered. For example, in a study of breast cancer survival in women who are grouped by age, 19–39, 40–69 and 70+, researchers might want to know whether survival decreases as age group increases. In other words is there a statistically significant negative association between the two measures? In these circumstances, they can use the *log-rank test for trend* (which again uses the chi-squared distribution). The null hypothesis is that there is no trend in survival across the ordered groups.

THE PROPORTIONAL HAZARDS (OR COX'S) REGRESSION MODEL

Although researchers can use the log-rank test to distinguish survival between two groups, the test only provides a p-value; it would be more useful to have an estimate of any difference in survival, along with the corresponding confidence interval. In addition, the test doesn't allow for adjustment for possible confounding variables, which may significantly affect survival. For this reason clinical papers will often contain the results of an approach known as *proportional hazards (or Cox's) regression*. This procedure will provide both estimates and confidence intervals for variables that affect survival and enable researchers to adjust for confounders. To improve your understanding of such material we will discuss briefly the principle underlying the method and the meaning of some of the terms you may encounter. The focus of *proportional hazards regression* is the *hazard*. The hazard is akin to a failure rate. If the end-point is death, for example, then the hazard is the rate at which individuals die at some point during the course of a study. The hazard can go up or down over time, and the distribution of hazards over the length of a study is known as the *hazard function*. You won't see authors quote the hazard regression function or equation but for those interested it looks like this:

$$\text{Hazard} = h_0 + e^{(\beta_1 X_1 + \beta_2 X_2 + \ldots)}$$

h_0 is the baseline hazard and is of little importance. The explanatory or independent variables can be any mixture of nominal, ordinal, or metric, and nominal variables can be 'dummied', as described previously. The same variable selection procedures as in linear or logistic regression models, i.e. automated or by hand, can also be used.

The most interesting property of this model is that e^{β_1}, e^{β_2}, etc. give us the *hazard ratios*, or HRs, for the variables X_1, X_2 and so on (notice the obvious similarity with the odds ratios in logistic regression). The hazard ratios are effectively *risk ratios*, but usually (although not always) referred to as hazard ratios in the context of survival studies (see also p. 133). So if X_1 is the 'Presence of micrometastases, Yes/No', (see Figure 27.2), then HR_1 is the hazard or risk of death for a patient when micrometastases are present compared to when they are absent. All of this is true only if the relative effect (essentially the *ratio*) of the hazard on the two groups (for example, the relative effect of micrometastases on the survival of each group), remains constant over the whole course of the study. Authors should show that they have checked the assumption of proportional hazard for each variable in the model (but rarely do so).

As an example of proportional hazards regression, Figure 27.4 is taken from a study into the relative survival of two groups of patients with non-metastatic colon cancer, one group having laparoscopy-assisted colectomy, the other open colectomy, (we also looked at this study in Chapter 21 in the context

Laparoscopy-assisted colectomy versus open colectomy for treatment of non-metastatic colon cancer: a randomised trial

Antonio M Lacy, Juan C Garcia-Valdecasas, Salvadora Delgado, Antoni Castells, Pilar Taura, Joseph M Pique, Joseph Visa

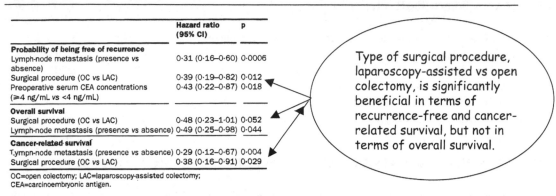

	Hazard ratio (95% CI)	p
Probability of being free of recurrence		
Lymph-node metastasis (presence vs absence)	0·31 (0·16–0·60)	0·0006
Surgical procedure (OC vs LAC)	0·39 (0·19–0·82)	0·012
Preoperative serum CEA concentrations (≥4 ng/mL vs <4 ng/mL)	0·43 (0·22–0·87)	0·018
Overall survival		
Surgical procedure (OC vs LAC)	0·48 (0·23–1·01)	0·052
Lymph-node metastasis (presence vs absence)	0·49 (0·25–0·98)	0·044
Cancer-related survival		
Lympn-node metastasis (presence vs absence)	0·29 (0·12–0·67)	0·004
Surgical procedure (OC vs LAC)	0·38 (0·16–0·91)	0·029

OC=open colectomy; LAC=laparoscopy-assisted colectomy;
CEA=carcinoembryonic antigen.

Type of surgical procedure, laparoscopy-assisted vs open colectomy, is significantly beneficial in terms of recurrence-free and cancer-related survival, but not in terms of overall survival.

FIGURE 27.4 Results of a Cox proportional hazards regression analysis comparing the survival of patients with laparoscopy-assisted colectomy versus open colectomy for the treatment of non-metastatic colon cancer

of the two-sample *t*-test, see Figure 21.6). Figure 27.4 shows the hazard ratios and confidence intervals for the probability of being free of recurrence, for overall survival, and for cancer-related survival, after the patients were stratified according to tumour stage.

So, for example, patients with lymph-node metastasis do only about a third as well in terms of being recurrence-free over the course of the study compared to patients without lymph-node metastasis (hazard ratio = 0.31), and this difference is statistically significant since the confidence interval does not include 1 (and the *p*-value of 0.0006 is <0.05). Patients with lymph-node metastasis also compare badly with non-metastasis patients in terms of both overall survival (only about a half as well, HR = 0.49), and cancer-related survival (just over a quarter as well, HR = 0.29), respectively. Both these results are statistically significant. Note that type of surgery, laparoscopy-assisted versus open colectomy, is not statistically significant in terms of overall survival, the confidence interval, (0.23–1.01), includes 1. However laparoscopy-assisted colectomy has significantly greater benefit than open colectomy for being recurrence-free and for cancer-related survival; 61% less chance of reoccurrence and 62% less chance of cancer-related death, respectively.

Checking the proportional hazards assumption

The proportional hazards assumption can be checked graphically using what is known as the *log-log* plot. You will sometimes find authors mentioning that they have carried out this check. For example, Freedland *et al.* (2005), in a study of prostate cancer survival after radical prostatectomy, write that:

> "The proportional hazards assumption of the Cox model was tested through the graphical examination of the log-log plots of the variables used in the model. These plots formed approximate paralleled lines as required."

Unfortunately we do not have the space to discuss this or other procedures any further; interested readers should refer to Hosmer and Lemeshow (1999).

VIII

Reading Between the Lines: How Authors Use Text, Tables and Pictures to Tell You What They've Done

28

Results in Text and Tables

RAW RESULTS AND COOKED FINDINGS

Study results are often set out in three stages: first, the raw *results*; second, the selection and summary of results into *findings*; and third the interpretation of these findings to produce *conclusions* (conclusions are dealt with in Chapter 30). Often some raw results and the consequent findings are presented in the text. Another strategy is to present raw results in tables, with the text extracting the findings that the authors reckon to be the key points (see Figure 28.1).

Equally often, raw results are displayed in tables but analysed further before being written out again in the text as summarized findings. In the next example, from a study of bleeding from the upper gastrointestinal tract, the text and table set out raw results in some detail, but the text goes on to make selected key points after applying further calculations (see Figure 28.2).

INTERESTING FINDINGS

Many of the most interesting findings from research investigations are those arising from comparisons between two (or more) groups of subjects. Notice in the text of Figure 28.2 that the authors have calculated and drawn our attention to higher incidences of bleeding and greater mortality among older people, and in men compared with women. In setting out these kinds of comparisons, researchers often employ two technical devices. First, they tell us the findings accompanied by the statistical estimations of confidence intervals and/or hypothesis tests (described in Chapters 18–20). Second (although not applied to the data in Figure 28.2), they may express their comparisons in terms of the kinds of fractions and ratios described in Chapters 16–18. To comprehend the findings of many papers you will need to be comfortable with risk ratios (relative risk) and odds ratios (Chapter 18), and the confidence intervals for each (Chapter 20). Risk ratios are typically used to describe the findings of cohort studies and clinical trials, while odds ratios are applied to case–control studies. There has been recently an unfortunate fad for the use of odds ratios in reporting clinical trials. It is not incorrect to summarize trial findings as odds ratios but it is difficult to interpret their meaning. Almost everyone finds risk ratios easier to translate into the everyday parlance of chance: such as, 'twice the chance of recovery in one group compared with the other'. The next two figures are illustrations of typical reporting of risk ratios (here called relative risk) (Figure 28.3) and odds ratios (Figure 28.4).

LEGENDS AND BRACKETS

Tables can be difficult to follow – not surprising when many contain a great deal of information. But even simple tables are hard to understand if they are not well set out and labelled with care. A table should bear a clear description of what it contains, together with a guide to its components – often called its *legend*.

Understanding Clinical Papers Second Edition   David Bowers, Allan House, David Owens
© 2006 John Wiley & Sons, Ltd

Prevalence of serious eye disease and visual impairment in a north London population: population based, cross sectional study

A Reidy, D C Minassian, G Vafidis, J Joseph, S Farrow, J Wu, P Desai, A Connolly

Results

The survey was carried out from April 1995 to October 1996, and 1547 people were examined and included in the sample. Of these, 1459 (94.3%) were white. Age and sex distribution in the sample was similar to that of the population of the area sampled (figure on website).

Response rate

The overall response rate was 1547/1840 (84% of those invited to participate). This was achieved after up to three rounds of invitation to attend. Non-responders were similar to respondents in terms of age, sex, and attending hospital clinics or opticians. Not having access to a telephone at home was more common in non-responders and in those who had to be re-invited for the third time.

Population prevalence of eye disorders

Table 1 shows that the population prevalence of visual impairment caused by cataract was 30%, that caused by age related macular degeneration was 8%, and that caused by refractive error was 9%. The prevalence of chronic open angle glaucoma was 3%, and a further 7% of subjects were suspected of having glaucoma. Table 2 shows that impaired vision in one or both eyes, present in more than half of the sample (815/1547), was potentially remediable in 69% of cases.

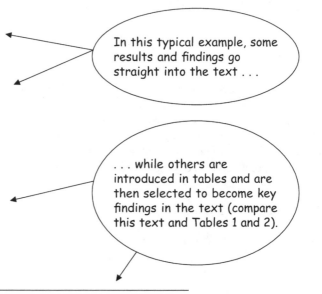

In this typical example, some results and findings go straight into the text . . .

. . . while others are introduced in tables and are then selected to become key findings in the text (compare this text and Tables 1 and 2).

Notice how the precision of the results is estimated using confidence intervals.

Table 1 Population prevalence (%) of main eye disorders

Eye disorders	No of cases in sample	Estimated population prevalence (95% CI)*	Estimated No of cases in population of 13 371 (95% CI)*
Cataract (lens opacity; one or both eyes; visual acuity <6/12)	451	30 (25.1 to 35.3)	4037 (3351 to 4723)
Had cataract surgery (one or both eyes)	162	10 (8.5 to 12.4)	1399 (1141 to 1657)
Age related macular degeneration (visual acuity <6/12)	133	8 (5.8 to 10.8)	1108 (776 to 1440)
Glaucoma (chronic open angle)	47	3 (2.3 to 3.6)	395 (306 to 485)
Suspected glaucoma	109	7 (5.4 to 8.4)	924 (719 to 1128)
Refractive error causing visual impairment one or both eyes; visual acuity <6/12	136	9 (7.0 to 11.4)	1228 (935 to 1521)

*Weighted average of cluster specific prevalence measures; calculations take into account the two stage cluster random sampling design.

Table 2 Visual impairment in the population and the proportion likely to be remediable through surgery or refraction and dispensing of spectacles

Visual impairment or blindness (visual acuity <6/12)	Estimated population prevalence (%) (95% CI)*	No of cases in sample[†]	Proportion (%) potentially remediable
One eye only	23.6 (20.9 to 26.3)	367	65
Both eyes	30.2 (24.8 to 35.5)	448	72
Total	53.8 (48.4 to 59.2)	815	69

*Weighted average of cluster specific prevalence measures; calculations take into account the two stage cluster random sampling design. [†]Eye disorders causing visual impairment: cataract, corneal opacity, posterior subcapsular opacity, and refractive error (including uncorrected aphakia or pseudophakia).

FIGURE 28.1   Extract from a results section to illustrate the interplay of text and tables

Acute upper gastrointestinal haemorrhage in west of Scotland: case ascertainment study

Oliver Blatchford, Lindsay A Davidson, William R Murray, Mary Blatchford, Jill Pell

Results

A total of 1882 adult cases were coded. This includes 61 patients whose acute upper gastrointestinal haemorrhage occurred while they were inpatients for other reasons and 61 patients who were transferred from other hospitals. Table 1 shows summary details of the patients' ages, sex distribution, and diagnoses.

In eight cases the final outcome of the episode was not recorded owing to incompleteness of the clinical record. No postcode could be traced in 24 cases, and the recorded postcodes were not valid in 52.

Incidence

The adult population of the area from which these patients were admitted was 2 184 285 at the 1991 census, giving an overall incidence of 172 per 100 000 people aged 15 and over per annum (95% confidence interval 165 to 180).

The incidence rose sharply with age, being 5.7 times higher among those over 75 than among those aged 15 to 29; P<0.00001), and it was twice as high among men as among women (P<0.00001). Table 1 also shows that the incidence of acute upper gastro-intestinal haemorrhage also rose with increasing Carstairs deprivation score, being 2.2 times greater in the most deprived quarter than in the most affluent quarter (P<0.00001).

Mortality

There were 153 deaths among the 1882 patients, resulting in an overall population mortality of 14.0 per 100 000 per annum (11.9 to 16.4). The population mortality increased sharply with increasing age (113 times greater among those over 75 than among those aged 15 to 29; P<0.00001) (table 1), and mortality among men was 1.6 times greater than among women (P=0.005). The population mortality in the most deprived quarter was double that in the least deprived quarter (P<0.0002).

> This section of the text shows raw results—details of sample size, inclusions and exclusions.

> This section of the text summarizes findings drawn from the preceding results in text and table—first applying additional calculations.

Table 1 Patient characteristics by incidence of and mortality and case fatality from acute upper gastrointestinal haemorrhage

	No of patients	Incidence (95% CI) (per 100 000 per year)	No of deaths	Mortality (95% CI) (per 100 000 per year)	Case fatality (%)
All cases	1882	172 (165 to 180)	153	14.0 (11.9 to 16.4)	8.1 (6.9 to 9.6)
Sex:					
Male	1208	236	89	17.4	7.4
Female	674	116	64	11	9.6
Statistics:					
Relative risk (95% CI) for women		0.49 (0.45 to 0.54)		0.63 (0.46 to 0.87)	1.29 (0.95 to 1.76)
χ^2 for trend (p value)		229 (<0.00001)		7.96 (0.005)	2.67 (0.1)
Age group (years):					
15–29	251	84	2	0.7	0.8
30–44	316	111	5	1.8	1.6
45–59	410	176	23	9.9	5.6
60–74	500	260	56	29.2	11.2
≥75	405	480	67	79.3	16.6
χ^2 for trend (p value)		635 (<0.00001)		261 (0.00001)	80 (<0.00001)
Deprivation score (quarters):*					
1 (most affluent)	316	114	27	9.7	9.4
2	389	144	20	7.4	5.4
3	433	159	45	16.5	11.6
4 (least affluent)	668	247	52	19.2	8.5
χ^2 for trend (p value)		141 (<0.00001)		14.6 (<0.0002)	0.24 (0.6)

*Excludes 76 cases in which deprivation score was missing.

> Notice that the text: (i) condenses raw table results (on age and deprivation) into clear statements about the findings; and (ii) describes further analysis of table results on incidence.

FIGURE 28.2 Extract from another results section to illustrate more complex interplay between text and tables

Mortality associated with oral contraceptive use: 25 year follow up of cohort of 46 000 women from Royal College of General Practitioners' oral contraception study

Valerie Beral, Carol Hermon, Clifford Kay, Philip Hannaford, Sarah Darby, Gillian Reeves

Abstract

Objective To describe the long term effects of the use of oral contraceptives on mortality.

Design Cohort study with 25 year follow up. Details of oral contraceptive use and of morbidity and mortality were reported six monthly by general practitioners. 75% of the original cohort was "flagged" on the NHS central registers.

Setting 1400 general practices throughout Britain.

Subjects 46 000 women, half of whom were using oral contraceptives at recruitment in 1968–9. Median age at end of follow up was 49 years.

Main outcome measures Relative risks of death adjusted for age, parity, social class, and smoking.

Results Over the 25 year follow up 1599 deaths were reported. Over the entire period of follow up the risk of death from all causes was similar in ever users and never users of oral contraceptives (relative risk=1.0, 95% confidence interval 0.9 to 1.1; P=0.7) and the risk of death for most specific causes did not differ significantly in the two groups. However, among current and recent (within 10 years) users the relative risk of death from ovarian cancer was 0.2 (0.1 to 0.8; P=0.01), from cervical cancer 2.5 (1.1 to 6.1; P=0.04), and from cerebrovascular disease 1.9 (1.2 to 3.1, P=0.009). By contrast, for women who had stopped use ≥10 years previously there were no significant excesses or deficits either overall or for any specific cause of death.

> Remember that a relative risk (risk ratio) of 1 indicates the same risk in each group; hence the statement here that death from all causes was as likely among users and non-users.

> The way these findings are worded, a relative risk below 1 suggests less risk of ovarian cancer among pill users.
>
> A relative risk above 1 suggests greater risk of cervical cancer among pill users.

FIGURE 28.3 The display of risk ratios (relative risk) to summarize findings from a cohort study

We find the legend of the table in Figure 28.5 a model of clarity. It is taken from a randomized controlled trial that compared routine general practitioner care with the effect of putting the patient in touch with a facilitator (from the 'Amalthea Project') whose task was to facilitate contact with relevant voluntary organisations. Study subjects were patients whose general practitioner thought they had psychosocial problems well suited to voluntary sector assistance. The table legend sets out first what the table contains – baseline characteristics of the subjects at the start of the study. Second, it tells us what the numerical values indicate – in this case, numbers of subjects unless stated otherwise. Third, it tells the reader what the brackets contain (percentages).

Risk factors for erysipelas of the leg (cellulitis): case-control study

Alain Dupuy, Hakima Benchikhi, Jean-Claude Roujeau, Philippe Bernard, Loïc Vaillant, Oliver Chosidow, Bruno Sassolas, Jean-Claude Guillaume, Jean-Jacques Grob, Sylvie Bastuji-Garin

Abstract

Objective To assess risk factors for erysipelas of the leg (cellulitis).
Design Case-control study.
Setting 7 hospital centres in France.
Subjects 167 patients admitted to hospital for erysipelas of the leg and 294 controls.
Results In multivariate analysis, a disruption of the cutaneous barrier (leg ulcer, wound, fissurated toe-web intertrigo, pressure ulcer, or leg dermatosis) (odds ratio 23.8, 95% confidence interval 10.7 to 52.5), lymphoedema (71.2, 5.6 to 908), venous insufficiency (2.0, 1.0 to 8.7), leg oedema (2.5, 1.2 to 5.1) and being overweight (2.0, 1.1 to 3.7) were independently associated with erysipelas of the leg. No association was observed with diabetes, alcohol, or smoking. Population attributable risk for toe-web intertrigo was 61%.
Conclusion This first case-control study highlights the major role of local risk factors (mainly lymphoedema and site of entry) in erysipelas of the leg. From a public health perspective, detecting and treating toe-web intertrigo should be evaluated in the secondary prevention of erysipelas of the leg.

Just as with the risk ratio, when the odds ratio is 1, it signifies that odds are the same in each group.

All the odds ratios here are greater than 1—suggesting greater risk of cellulitis in those with each characteristic. In particular, it looks like broken skin or lymphoedema are especially prevalent among cellulitis sufferers.

FIGURE 28.4   The display of odds ratios to summarize findings from a case–control study

DASHES

Brackets cause confusion when the legend doesn't tell you what is in them. Dashes are even more hazardous: the problem is that we use the same device – a dash – to indicate range and as a minus sign. Here are extracts from two further tables from the same study (Figure 28.6). It is self-evident that the dashes in their *Table 5* are being used to indicate range. You may find it less obvious that the dashes in their *Table 4* indicate minus signs. The legend for Table 4 tells us that the first column of values refers to *differences* in various measures before and after the study interventions. A minus difference on the scales shown here indicates improvement (less anxiety, for example).

Displaying confidence intervals requires particular care (see Chapter 19). The interval might reasonably be written, for example, as (4–9). But recall that when confidence intervals express the range around a difference between two proportions or between two means, then one or both of the confidence limits often has a minus sign. No wonder then that it is sensible always to write the interval as something like (4 to 9) or (−4 to 9) to prevent ambiguity. In Table 5 in Figure 28.6 there are lots of minus signs, so it's a mercy that the intervals are consistently written as one value *to* another. Not all authors or journals are as careful about this simple safeguard as in the examples here, so watch out for dashes.

A randomised controlled trial and economic evaluation of a referrals facilitator between primary care and the voluntary sector

Clare Grant, Trudy Goodenough, Ian Harvey, Chris Hine

Table 1 Characteristics of patients at baseline. Values are numbers (percentages) unless stated otherwise

Characteristic	Amalthea group (n=90)	General practitioner group (n=71)
Sex:		
Male	65 (72)	56 (79)
Female	25 (28)	15 (21)
Mean (SD) age in years (range):		
All patients	40.8 (15.5, 17–86)	45.6 (16.8, 18–86)
Marital status:		
Single	23 (26)	14 (22)
Married or cohabiting	40 (44)	29 (45)
Widowed	7 (8)	7 (11)
Divorced or separated	20 (22)	14 (22)
Data missing	0	7
Social class:		
I and II	13 (15)	11 (18)
III manual and non manual	22 (25)	15 (25)
IV and V	9 (10)	4 (7)
Economically inactive	44 (50)	31 (51)
Data missing	2	10
History of mental illness:		
Yes	18 (24)	12 (25)
Data missing	16	22

Notice that when the values stop being numbers of subjects but means (with standard deviations and ranges in brackets), this alteration is easy to follow because of the clear legend.

Notice also how the indentation is used to clarify meaning: 'data missing' appears three times but it is always evident which data are missing—marital status, social class, or history of mental illness.

FIGURE 28.5 How the clarity of a table depends on its layout and the legend

The last table in this chapter (Figure 28.7) has been included to show how authors and journal editorial staff, by liberal but careful use of brackets, dashes and to's, can successfully and economically display a lot of different kinds of results yet avoid confusing the reader. Despite their efforts they don't always achieve final products as clear as this one and the earlier tables shown in this section.

A randomised controlled trial and economic evaluation of a referrals facilitator between primary care and the voluntary sector

Clare Grant, Trudy Goodenough, Ian Harvey, Chris Hine

Table 4 Difference between outcome measure scores of patients in two arms of trial from repeated measures analysis of covariance after adjustment for baseline score

Outcome measure	Differences for combined follow up period (95% CI)	P value
Hospital anxiety and depression scale		
Anxiety	−1.9 (−3.0 to −0.7)	0.002
Depression	−0.9 (−1.9 to 0.2)	0.116
DUKE-UNC functional social support scale		
Confidant support	−0.9 (−2.4 to 0.6)	0.221
Affective support	−0.3 (−1.2 to 0.7)	0.594

In all the values here, the dash is a minus sign, so the word 'to' is used to indicate range.

Table 5 Mean and range of resource utilisation for patients in two arms of trial

Outcome measure	Amalthea group (n=89)*	General practitioner group (n=68)†
No of contacts with primary healthcare team	4.4 (1–13)	4.4 (1–13)
Cost of contacts with primary healthcare team (£)	61 (14–188)	69 (9–202)
No of prescriptions	3.2 (0–30)	2.0 (0–16)
No of mental health prescriptions	1.9 (0–30)	0.9 (0–8)
Cost of prescriptions (£)	25 (0–169)	22 (0–209)
No of referrals	0.3 (0–2)	0.5 (0–4)
No of mental health referrals	0.2 (0–2)	0.3 (0–2)
Cost of referrals (£)	21 (0–146)	42 (0–322)
Total cost of primary healthcare team contacts, prescribing, and referrals (£)	107 (14–340)	133 (10–452)

(1-13) obviously indicates a range between 1 and 13.

FIGURE 28.6   Extracts from tables, illustrating the two common ways of using dashes

Patient satisfaction with outpatient hysteroscopy versus day care hysteroscopy: randomised controlled trial

Christian Kremer, Sean Duffy, Michelle Moroney

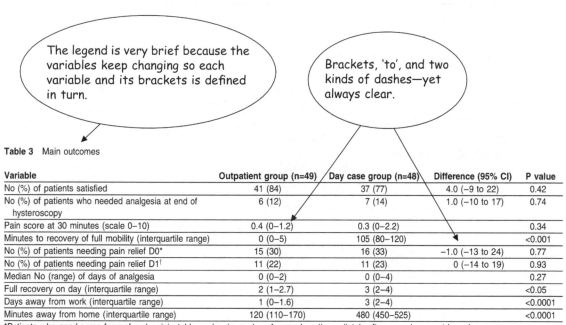

The legend is very brief because the variables keep changing so each variable and its brackets is defined in turn.

Brackets, 'to', and two kinds of dashes—yet always clear.

Table 3 Main outcomes

Variable	Outpatient group (n=49)	Day case group (n=48)	Difference (95% CI)	P value
No (%) of patients satisfied	41 (84)	37 (77)	4.0 (−9 to 22)	0.42
No (%) of patients who needed analgesia at end of hysteroscopy	6 (12)	7 (14)	1.0 (−10 to 17)	0.74
Pain score at 30 minutes (scale 0–10)	0.4 (0–1.2)	0.3 (0–2.2)		0.34
Minutes to recovery of full mobility (interquartile range)	0 (0–5)	105 (80–120)		<0.001
No (%) of patients needing pain relief D0*	15 (30)	16 (33)	−1.0 (−13 to 24)	0.77
No (%) of patients needing pain relief D1†	11 (22)	11 (23)	0 (−14 to 19)	0.93
Median No (range) of days of analgesia	0 (0–2)	0 (0–4)		0.27
Full recovery on day (interquartile range)	2 (1–2.7)	3 (2–4)		<0.05
Days away from work (interquartile range)	1 (0–1.6)	3 (2–4)		<0.0001
Minutes away from home (interquartile range)	120 (110–170)	480 (450–525)		<0.0001

*Patients who need some form of oral or injectable analgesia on day of procedure (immediately after procedure or at home).
†Patients who need some form of oral or injectable analgesia on day after procedure.

FIGURE 28.7 A table that successfully uses brackets, dashes and the word 'to'

29

Results in Pictures

WHY USE CHARTS AND FIGURES?

Research authors and journal publishers generally do their best to make sure that the display of figures is informative and economical of space, so that 'A picture paints a thousand words'. There are two ways that research figures can achieve these aims: by displaying data graphically when they cannot readily be shown another way; and by using the figure to create a striking impact – even when the findings might effectively have been placed within text or tables. Of course these aims are not consistently met, and sometimes the publisher's main aim in printing charts and figures may be to break up large blocks of unattractive text and tables.

Figure 29.1 is an example of a chart which shows how the study data, in two groups of subjects, are derived from all the people who might possibly have been subjects. It's hard to imagine how the information here could be presented as clearly and concisely as text or in a table.

The next example (Figure 29.2) is one where the data might readily have been placed in either text or table but the impact of the picture is intended to demonstrate how the whole is divided into proportions. Pie charts work to show the parts of a whole, so comparisons between two or more groups can be displayed only by placing multiple pies side by side. Bar charts, on the other hand, lend themselves to the comparison of two or more groups, all in one figure. The apparently simple chart in Figure 29.3 has considerable impact, displaying a striking reduction in the tropical eye disease trachoma after fly control in villages in The Gambia. On closer inspection, though, it is surprisingly complex – comparing villages that were sprayed with those that were not, in two seasons of the year, in each case measuring trachoma prevalence twice. You will need to concentrate to comprehend the story behind the data; we think that neither text nor table could readily present the findings as clearly or economically.

There are a great many additions and refinements to the basic bar chart. One extra you will often encounter is a line, often known as an *error bar*, sticking out of and penetrating into the main bar, as in Figure 29.4. The authors are using the error bars to illustrate how precisely the main bars estimate the population values (see Chapter 19). In general, authors use either the standard error or the 95% confidence interval; they should tell you which one (but often they forget to). Neither is particularly to be preferred to the other. Less often, the error bar may be a standard deviation (see Chapter 12), which is rarely if ever helpful on a bar chart.

Sometimes you will see a line graph instead of a bar chart – particularly when the horizontal axis is *time*. When there are two or more samples being compared, the effect of joining up the points for each sample shows the pattern over time rather better than would a comparable bar chart (Figure 29.5). Error bars are often included with line graphs and fulfil much the same function as they do with bars.

Another trimming sometimes added to the bar chart is the splitting of the bars into subdivisions, giving the feel of bars stacked on top of one another. The advantage of economy of information is countered by a problem with visual interpretation because only the lowest part of the bar has a fixed baseline, so the pattern of the higher parts of the bars can easily be missed. In the fairly typical example shown here as Figure 29.6 the patterns evident in the lowest part of the bars are the easiest to grasp.

The layout of a bar chart suggests some content to the area of each bar – between the baseline and the limit of the bar – often used to display values for proportions or means. When the value to be displayed

Understanding Clinical Papers Second Edition   David Bowers, Allan House, David Owens
© 2006 John Wiley & Sons, Ltd

Intensity of leg and arm training after primary middle-cerebral-artery stroke: a randomised trial

Gert Kwakkel, Robert C Wagenaar, Jos W R Twisk, Gustaaf J Lankhorst, Johan C Koetsier

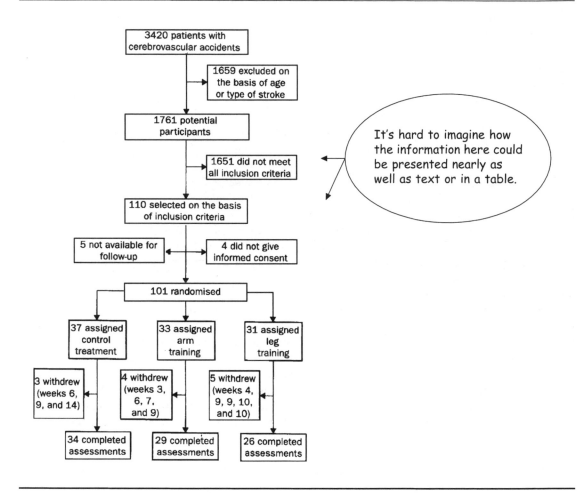

FIGURE 29.1 Trial profile: showing what happened to all potentially eligible subjects

is an odds ratio or a risk ratio, then there is no baseline and consequently no substance to any of the space. Consequently, values for risk ratios or odds ratios are often, as in Figure 29.7, marked on the chart with no bar to be seen.

SHAPE OF DISTRIBUTIONS

Histograms show a distributed, metric variable chopped up into equal sized bands – such that the shape of the accumulated bars accurately displays the *shape* of the data (see Chapter 11). In the example in

Effect of metoprolol CR/XL in chronic heart failure: Metoprolol CR/XL Randomised Intervention Trial in Congestive Heart Failure (MERIT-HF)

MERIT-HF Study Group

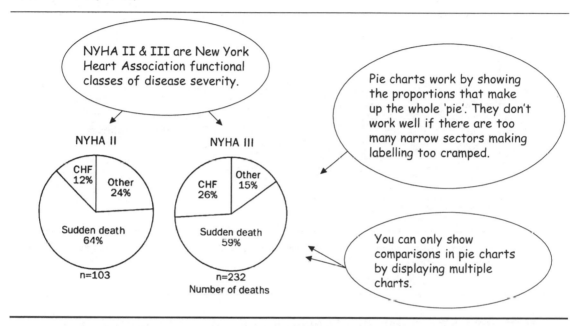

FIGURE 29.2 Pie charts showing severity of heart failure and mode of death

Figure 29.8, the graph shape shows that there was over-representation of older people among the sample of patients who had experienced pulmonary emboli. Although bar charts are drawn with gaps between bars, histograms keep the whole data set together without gaps.

When data are skewed, or when the data are ordinal categorical (see Chapter 11), researchers may choose to present the distribution graphically using a box plot (or box-and-whisker chart). The example in Figure 29.9 explains how these pictures are constructed. They use the rank order measures of spread that were set out in Chapter 12.

Effect of fly control on trachoma and diarrhoea

Paul M Emerson, Steve W Lindsay, Gijs E L Walraven, Hannah Faal, Claus Bøgh, Kebba Lowe, Robin L Bailey

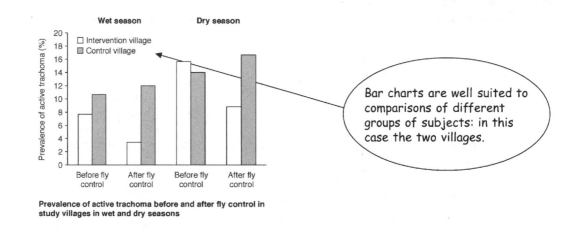

Prevalence of active trachoma before and after fly control in study villages in wet and dry seasons

FIGURE 29.3 Bar chart comparing disease prevalence before and after fly control in control and intervention study villages in wet and dry seasons

Quantitative assessment of cervical spondylotic myelopathy by a simple walking test

Anoushka Singh, H Alan Crockard

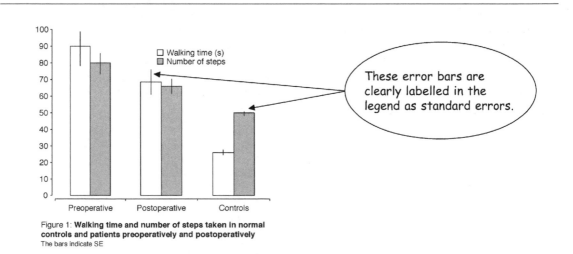

Figure 1: **Walking time and number of steps taken in normal controls and patients preoperatively and postoperatively**
The bars indicate SE

FIGURE 29.4 Bar chart with error bars

Comparison of combination therapy with single-drug therapy in early rheumatoid arthritis: a randomised trial

Timo Möttönen, Pekka Hannonen, Marjatta Leirisalo-Repo, Martti Nissilä, Hannu Kautianinen, Markku Korpela, Leena Laasonen, Heikki Julkunen, Raijo Luukkainen, Kaisa Vuori, Leena Paimela, Harri Bläfield, Markku Hakala, Kirsti Ilva, Urpo Yli-Kerttula, Kari Puolakka, Pentti Järvinen, Mikko Hakola, Heikki Piirainen, Jari Ahonen, Ilppo Pälvimäki, Sinikka Forsberg, Kalevi Koota, Claes Friman, for the FIN-RACo trial group*

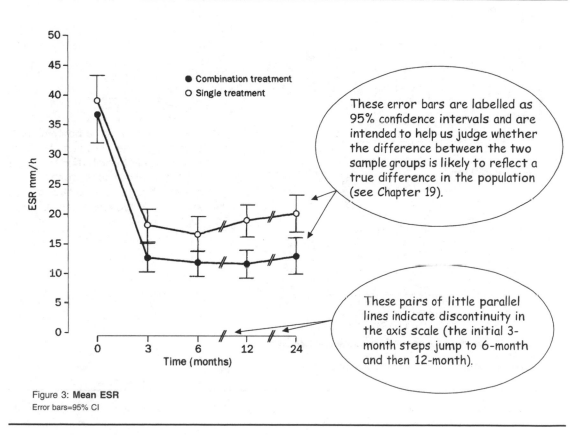

Figure 3: **Mean ESR**
Error bars=95% CI

FIGURE 29.5 Line graph of mean erythrocyte sedimentation rate (ESR) over two years of follow-up, showing ESR for single and combination treatment groups

Clinical progression and virological failure on highly active antiretroviral therapy in HIV-1 patients: a prospective cohort study

Bruno Ledergerber, Matthias Egger, Milos Opravil, Amalio Telenti, Bernard Hirschel, Manuel Battegay, Pietro Vernazza, Philippe Sudre, Markus Flepp, Hansjakob Furrer, Patrick Francioli, Rainer Weber, for the Swiss HIV Cohort Study*

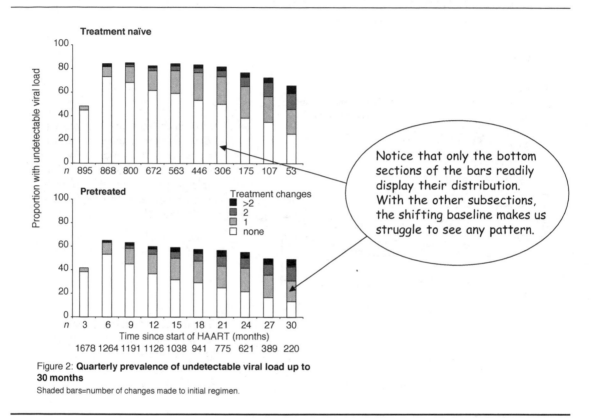

Figure 2: **Quarterly prevalence of undetectable viral load up to 30 months**

Shaded bars=number of changes made to initial regimen.

FIGURE 29.6 Stacked bar charts displaying time pattern of undetectable viral load for four subdivisions of the sample according to number of treatment changes

Factors influencing the effect of age on prognosis in breast cancer: population based study

Niels Kroman, Maj-Britt Jensen, Jan Wohlfahrt, Henning T Mouridsen, Per Kragh Andersen, Mads Melbye

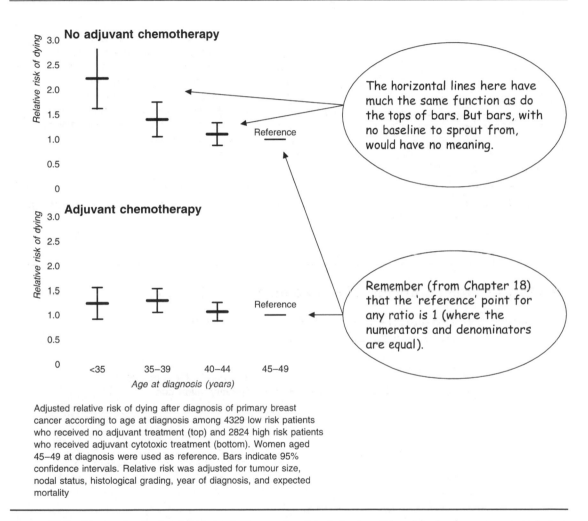

Adjusted relative risk of dying after diagnosis of primary breast cancer according to age at diagnosis among 4329 low risk patients who received no adjuvant treatment (top) and 2824 high risk patients who received adjuvant cytotoxic treatment (bottom). Women aged 45–49 at diagnosis were used as reference. Bars indicate 95% confidence intervals. Relative risk was adjusted for tumour size, nodal status, histological grading, year of diagnosis, and expected mortality

FIGURE 29.7   Chart using horizontal marks (with error bars) to indicate relative risks for four age groups in two cohorts who received or did not receive adjuvant chemotherapy for the treatment of breast cancer

Acute pulmonary embolism: clinical outcomes in the International Cooperative Pulmonary Embolism Registry (ICOPER)

Samuel Z Goldhaber, Luigi Visani, Marisa De Rosa, for ICOPER*

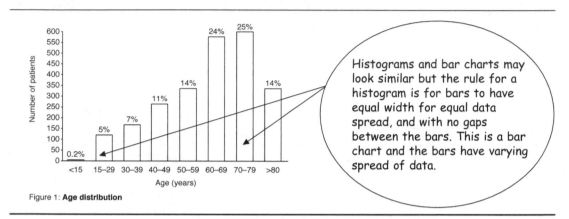

Figure 1: **Age distribution**

FIGURE 29.8   Bar chart of age distribution of 2454 consecutive patients with acute pulmonary embolism, drawn from 52 hospitals in seven countries

Decline in total serum IgE after treatment for tuberculosis

J F A Adams, E H Schölvinck, R P Gie, P C Potter, N Beyers, A D Beyers

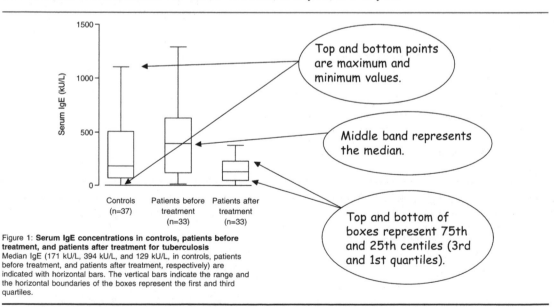

Figure 1: **Serum IgE concentrations in controls, patients before treatment, and patients after treatment for tuberculosis**
Median IgE (171 kU/L, 394 kU/L, and 129 kU/L, in controls, patients before treatment, and patients after treatment, respectively) are indicated with horizontal bars. The vertical bars indicate the range and the horizontal boundaries of the boxes represent the first and third quartiles.

FIGURE 29.9   A comparison of three box plots (or box-and-whisker charts), accompanied by a description of the conventional layout of the box plot

30

The Discussion and the Conclusions

The discussion section of a paper comes usually at the end, after the presentation of results, and is meant to put those results in context for the reader – indicating the authors' beliefs about the meaning of their findings and their implications for the future.

The discussion varies considerably in content and length, according to the style of the journal, but it is likely to contain some or all of the following elements. Discussions often start with a brief summary of the main findings of the study, as in Figure 30.1. This summary will usually contain little or no data or statistics – its purpose is to 'remind' you of the main message the authors would like you to take from their paper. It should certainly contain no new data, which always belong in the results section.

The findings may then be compared with those from other similar work, to point out whether they broadly agree with previous research or whether they disagree. This business of comparing findings with others can be difficult, mainly because it is so hard to get an accurate unbiased view of the previous research in an area. We tend to know certain papers well – especially if we have enjoyed them or they support our own views – and yet be unaware of other equally-important work. The best approach would be to refer to a *systematic review* of the literature (see Chapter 26), but one may not exist. If one doesn't (or it isn't quoted by the authors) then be cautious about the possibilities of bias from selective quotation in this mini-review.

Good discussions include a brief *critical appraisal* of the work that is presented: pointing out the main strengths *and weaknesses* of the study, and considering whether the results could have been due to some flaw in its design or conduct. A typical example is shown in Figure 30.2.

So far in the discussion, the authors should have reminded you of what their findings are and where they fit in to the total picture, and they should have indicated the likelihood that their results are believable and not due to problems with the study. In the next section you may find a suggestion as to the meaning of the findings: is there a plausible explanation for them? Any reader of crime or thriller novels knows that a plausible story may not turn out to be a true one, but nonetheless this is a useful exercise. If results fly in the face of everything we know, they may present an exciting challenge to our theories, but we are more likely to think twice about whether they are reliable. Journals (and authors) vary considerably in how much they like to explore this side of the work – 'getting away from the data' – and some discussions can seem too much like reviews in their own right.

The other way to discuss the meaning of results is to ask what their implications are for future practice. In clinical practice, the question is: 'If we believe these results, should it change how we work, and if so how?' Incidentally, this is a very good question to ask of yourself to decide if you *do* really believe the results, and if you really base your practice on evidence! Of course, answers are rarely clear-cut, and the other question to ask of the future is: 'What research do we need to do to build on the findings from this study, or to answer the questions raised by it?'

A few papers finish with a 'conclusions' or 'summary' section, but for most the abstract and discussion serve those purposes. Journals often have boxes (see Figure 30.3) or bullet-point lists to tell you about a paper. They can help you with a quick summary of what a paper is about, and they tell you what the authors would like to conclude from their study.

Understanding Clinical Papers Second Edition   David Bowers, Allan House, David Owens
© 2006 John Wiley & Sons, Ltd

A Nationwide Study of Decisions to Forgo Life-Prolonging Treatment in Dutch Medical Practice

Johanna H. Groenewoud, MD; Agnes van der Heide, MD, PhD; John G. C. Kester, MA; Carmen L. M. de Graaff, MA; Gerrit van der Wal, MC, PhD; Paul J. van der Maas, MD, PhD

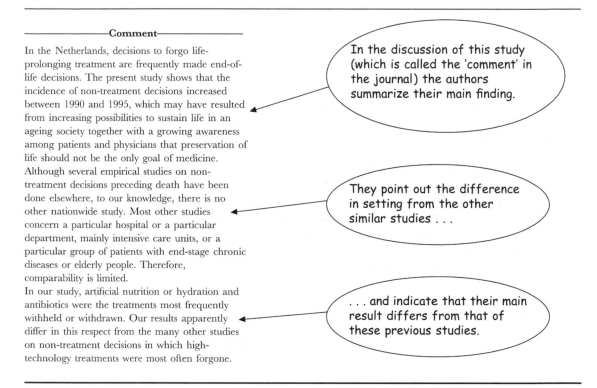

—————————Comment—————————

In the Netherlands, decisions to forgo life-prolonging treatment are frequently made end-of-life decisions. The present study shows that the incidence of non-treatment decisions increased between 1990 and 1995, which may have resulted from increasing possibilities to sustain life in an ageing society together with a growing awareness among patients and physicians that preservation of life should not be the only goal of medicine. Although several empirical studies on non-treatment decisions preceding death have been done elsewhere, to our knowledge, there is no other nationwide study. Most other studies concern a particular hospital or a particular department, mainly intensive care units, or a particular group of patients with end-stage chronic diseases or elderly people. Therefore, comparability is limited.

In our study, artificial nutrition or hydration and antibiotics were the treatments most frequently withheld or withdrawn. Our results apparently differ in this respect from the many other studies on non-treatment decisions in which high-technology treatments were most often forgone.

In the discussion of this study (which is called the 'comment' in the journal) the authors summarize their main finding.

They point out the difference in setting from the other similar studies . . .

. . . and indicate that their main result differs from that of these previous studies.

Figure 30.1 A discussion which starts with a résumé of the study findings

Crisis telephone consultation for deliberate self-harm patients: effects on repetition

Mark O Evans, H G Morgan, Alan Hayward and David J Gunnell

Discussion

Limitations of the study and representativeness of the sample population

Routine health service information systems were used to determine the proportion of patients who repeated DSH in the six month follow-up period. Such methods will underestimate repetition on three counts. First, subjects who migrate out of the study and/or who are admitted to hospitals other than the three study hospitals will not have repeat episodes detected. The fact that Bristol is a discrete urban area means that in practice this is likely to occur infrequently. Secondly, repeat acts of DSH not presenting to hospital but either managed by the general practitioner or by the patient alone without the help of secondary care services might not be identified. Thirdly, those patients repeating DSH by self-laceration (approximately 10% of all episodes) are less reliably detected. We have no reason to suspect that the above omissions will be distributed unevenly between the two arms of the trial.

The findings in this paper refer specifically to patients who were admitted to medical wards, hence the relatively large percentage of subjects with previous experience of DSH (48%) and the high rates of repeat DSH (16% in six months). Using routinely available data, we estimate that over the study period approximately 70% of DSH patients attending accident and emergency departments in Bristol were admitted to hospital (further details available

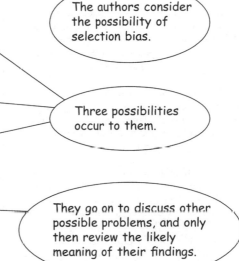

The authors consider the possibility of selection bias.

Three possibilities occur to them.

They go on to discuss other possible problems, and only then review the likely meaning of their findings.

FIGURE 30.2   Critical appraisal of a study's results

Risk of subarachnoid haemorrhage in first degree relatives of patients with subarachnoid haemorrhage: follow up study based on national registries in Denmark

Favid Gaist, Michael Vaeth, Ioannis Tsiropoulos, Kaare Christensen, Elisabeth Corder, Jørn Olsen, Henrik Toft Sørensen

What is known on this topic

Several observational studies have indicated that first degree relatives of patients with subarachnoid haemorrhage are at increased risk of having this disorder. However, the validity of the risk estimates could be questioned owing to potential problems of selection and recall bias.

What this paper adds

This follow up study overcame some of these problems by using national registries in Denmark to create pedigrees and to identify incident cases of subarachnoid haemorrhage.

The study confirmed that first degree relatives of patients with subarachnoid haemorrhage are at a threefold to fivefold increased risk of experiencing a subarachnoid haemorrhage compared with the general population but the incidence rate of subarachnoid haemorrhage is low.

Summary boxes like this will often appear near the end of a paper. They may help you decide whether the paper is likely to interest you, but you should never believe what they say without checking out the study for yourself.

FIGURE 30.3   A summary box which outlines a study's importance and main findings

References

Adams JFA, Schölvinck EH, Gie RP, Potter PC, Beyers N, Beyers AD. Decline in total serum IgE after treatment for tuberculosis. *Lancet* 1999, 353: 2030–2.

Adish AA, Esrey SA, Gyorkos TW, Jean-Baptiste J, Rojhani A. Effect of consumption of food cooked in iron pots on iron status and growth of young children: a randomised trial. *Lancet* 1999, 353: 712–16.

Altman D. *Practical Statistics for Medical Research*. London: Chapman and Hall, 1991.

Appleby L, Shaw J, Amos T, McDonnell R, Harris C, McCann K, Kiernan K, Davies S, Bickley H, Parsons R. Suicide within 12 months of contact with mental health services; national clinical survey. *BMJ* 1999, 318: 1235–9.

Appleby L, Warner R, Whitton A, Faragher B. A controlled study of fluoxetine and cognitive-behavioural counselling in the treatment of postnatal depression. *BMJ* 1997, 314: 932–5.

Basso O, Olsen J, Johansen AMT, Christensen K. Change in social status and risk of low birth weight in Denmark: population based cohort study. *BMJ* 1997, 315: 1498–502.

Beral V, Hermon C, Kay C, Hannaford P, Darby S, Reeves G. Mortality associated with oral contraceptive use: 25 year follow up of cohort of 46 000 women from Royal College of General Practitioners' oral contraception study. *BMJ* 1999, 318: 96–100.

Berkley J, Mwangi I, Griffiths K, Ahmed I, Mithwani S, EnglishM, Newton C, Maitland K. Assessment of severe malnutrition among hospitalised children in rural Kenya. *Journal of the American Medical Association* 2005, 294: 591–5.

Bhagwanjee S, Muckart DJJ, Jeena PM, Moodley P. Does HIV status influence the outcome of patients admitted to a surgical intensive care unit? A prospective double blind study. *BMJ* 1997, 314:1077.

Bland JM, Altman DG. Statistical methods for assessing agreement between two clinical measurements. *Lancet* 1986, i: 307–10.

Blatchford O, Davidson LA, Murray WR, Blatchford M, Pell J. Acute upper gastrointestinal haemorrhage in west of Scotland: case ascertainment study. *BMJ* 1997, 315: 510–14.

Bowers D. *Statistics from Scratch*. Chichester: John Wiley, 1996.

Bowling A (1997). *Research Methods in Health*. Maidenhead; Open University Press.

Brandon S, Cowley P, McDonald C, Neville P, Palmer R, Wellstood-Eason S. Electroconvulsive therapy: results in depressive illness from the Leicestershire trial. *BMJ* 1984, 288: 23–6.

Brent NB, Redd B, Dworetz A, D'Amico F, Greenberg JJ. Breast-feeding in a low-income population: program to increase incidence and duration. *Archives of Pediatrics and Adolescent Medicine* 1995, 149: 789–803.

Bruzzi P, Dogliotti L, Naldoni C, *et al.* Cohort study of association of risk of breast cancer with cyst type in women with gross cystic disease of the breast. *BMJ* 1997, 314: 925–8.

Carson AJ, Ringbauer B, MacKenzie L, Warlow C, Sharpe M. Neurological disease, emotional disorder, and disability: they are related. A study of 300 consecutive new referrals to a neurology outpatient department. *Journal of Neurology, Neurosurgery and Psychiatry* 2000; 68: 202–6.

Chosidow O, Chastang C, Brue C, Bouvet E, Izri M, Monteny N, Bastuji-Garin S, Rousset J-J, Revuz J. Controlled study of malathion and *d*-phenothrin lotions for *Pediculus humanus* var *capitis*-infected schoolchildren. *Lancet* 1994, 344: 1724–9.

Cooper JE, Goodhead D, Craig T, Harris M, Howat J, Korer J. The incidence of schizophrenia in Nottingham. *British Journal of Psychiatry* 1987, 151: 619–26.

Cooper KG, Bain C, Parkin DE. Comparison of microwave endometrial ablation and transcervical resection of the endometrium for treatment of heavy menstrual loss: a randomised trial. *Lancet* 1999, 354: 1859–63.

Coste J, Delecoeuillerie G, Cohen de Lara A, Le Parc JM, Paolaggi JB. Clinical course and prognostic factors in acute low back pain: an inception cohort study in primary care practice. *BMJ* 1994, 308: 577–80.

Understanding Clinical Papers Second Edition   David Bowers, Allan House, David Owens
© 2006 John Wiley & Sons, Ltd

Cousens SN, Zeidler M, Esmonde TF, De Silva R, Wilesmith JW, Smith PG, Will RG. Sporadic Creutzfeldt-Jakob disease in the United Kingdom: analysis of epidemiological surveillance data for 1970–96. *BMJ* 1997, 315: 389–95.

Criqui MH, Ringel BL. Does diet or alcohol explain the French paradox? *Lancet* 1994, 344: 1719–23.

Culbertson DS, Griggs M, Hudson S. Ear and hearing status in multilevel retirement facility. *Geriatric Nursing* 2004, 25: 93–6.

de Boer MA, Celentano DD, Tovanabutra S, Rugpao S, Nelson KE Suriyanon V. Reliability of self-reported sexual behaviour is human immunodeficiency virus (HIV) between concordant and discordant heterosexual couples in Northern Thailand. *American Journal of Epidemiology* 1998, 147: 1153–61.

Dunne MW, Bozzette S, McCutchan JA, Dubé MP, Sattler FR, Forthal D, Kemper CA, Havlir D, for the California Collaborative Treatment Group Efficacy of azithromycin in prevention of *Pneumocystis carinii* pneumonia: a randomised trial. *Lancet* 1999, 354: 891–4.

Dupuy A, Benchikhi H, Roujeau J-C, *et al*. Risk factors for erysipelas of the leg (cellulitis): case–control study. *BMJ* 1999, 318: 1591–4.

Egger M, Smith GD. Bias in location and selection of studies. *BMJ* 1998, 316: 61–6.

Ellenbecker CH, Frazier SC, Verney S. Nurses' observations and experiences of problems and adverse effects of medication management in home care. *Geriatric Nursing* 2004, 26: 164–70.

Emerson PM, Lindsay SW, Walraven GEL, *et al*. Effect of fly control on trachoma and diarrhoea. *Lancet* 1999, 353: 1401–3.

English RM, Badcock JC, Giay T, Ngu T, Waters A-M, Bennett SA. Effect of nutrition improvement project on morbidity from infectious diseases in preschool children in Vietnam: comparison with control commune, *BMJ* 1997, 315: 1122–5.

Evans MO, Morgan HG, Hayward A, Gunnell DJ. Crisis telephone consultation for deliberate self-harm patients: effects on repetition. *British Journal of Psychiatry* 1999, 175: 23–7.

Fahey T, Stocks N, Thomas T. Quantitative systematic review of randomised controlled trials comparing antibiotic with placebo for acute cough in adults. *BMJ* 1998, 316: 906–10.

Farnell S, Maxwell L, Tan S, Rhodes A, Philips B. Temperature measurement: comparison of non-invasive methods used in adult critical care. *Journal of Clinical Nursing* 2005, 14: 632–9.

Feeney M, Clegg A, Winwood P, Snook J. for the East Dorset Gastroenterology Group A case–control study of measles vaccination and inflammatory bowel disease. *Lancet* 1997, 350: 764–6.

Field A (2000) *Discovering Statistics Using SPSS for Windows*, London: Sage.

Gaist F, Vaeth M, Tsiropoulos I, Christensen K, Corder E, Olsen J, Toft Sørensen H. Risk of subarachnoid haemorrhage in first degree relatives of patients with subarachnoid haemorrhage: follow up study based on national registries in Denmark. *BMJ* 2000, 320: 141–5.

Gibbs S, Harvey I, Sterling JC, Stark R. Local treatment for cutaneous warts. *Cochrane Database of Systematic Reviews* 2005, 3.

Goldhaber SZ, Visani L, De Rosa M. Acute pulmonary embolism: clinical outcomes in the International Cooperative Pulmonary Embolism Registry (ICOPER). *Lancet* 1999, 353: 1386–9.

Graham W, Smith P, Kamal A, Fitzmaurice A, Smith N, Hamilton N. Randomised controlled trial comparing effectiveness of touch screen with leaflet for providing women with information on prenatal tests. *BMJ* 2000, 320: 155–60.

Grandjean P, Bjerve KS, Weihe P, Steuerwald U. Birthweight in a fishing community: significance of essential fatty acids and marine food contaminants. *International Journal of Epidemiology* 2000, 30: 1272–7.

Grant C, Goodenough T, Harvey I, Hine C. A randomised controlled trial and economic evaluation of a referrals facilitator between primary care and the voluntary sector. *BMJ* 2000, 320: 419–23.

Griffin S. Diabetes care in general practice: meta-analysis of randomised control trials. *BMJ* 1998, 317: 390–6.

Groenewoud JH, van der Heide A, Kester JGC, de Graaff CLM, van der Wal G, van der Maas PJ. A nationwide study of decisions to forgo life-prolonging treatment in Dutch medical practice. *Archives of Internal Medicine* 2000, 160: 357–63.

Grun L, Tassono-Smith J, Carder C, Johnson AM, Robinson A, Murray E, Stephenson J, Haines A, Copas A, Ridgway G. Comparison of two methods of screening for genital chlamydial infection in women attending in general practice: cross sectional survey. *BMJ* 1997, 315: 226–30.

Haelterman E, Bréart G, Paris-Llado J, Dramaix M, Tchobroutsky C. Effect of uncomplicated chronic hypertension on the risk of small-for-gestational age birth. *American Journal of Epidemiology* 1997, 145: 689–95.

Hagen S, Bugge C, Alexander H. Psychometric properties of the SF36 in the early post-stroke phase. *Journal of Advanced Nursing* 2003, 44: 461–8.

Hancox RJ, Milne BJ, Poulton R. Association between child and adolescent television viewing and adult health: a longitudinal birth cohort study, *Lancet* 2003, 364: 257–62.

Hawton K, Fagg J, Simkin S, Bale E, Bond A. Trends in deliberate self-harm in Oxford, 1985–1995: implications for the clinical services and the prevention of suicide. *British Journal of Psychiatry* 1997, 171: 556–60.

He Y, Lam TH, Li LS, Du RY, Jia GL, Huang JY, Zheng JS. Passive smoking at work as a risk factor for coronary heart disease in Chinese women who have never smoked. *BMJ* 1994, 308: 380–4.

Hearn J, Higinson IJ. Development and validation of a core outcome measure for palliative care: the palliative care outcome scale. *Quality in Health Care* 1999, 8: 219–27.

Henderson RD, Wliasziw M, Fox AJ, Rothwell PM, Barnett HJM, for the North American Symptomatic Carotid Endarterectomy Trial Group. Angiographically defined collateral circulation and risk of stroke in patients with severe carotid artery stenosis. *Stroke* 2000, 31: 128–32.

Ho Cheung W, Lopez V. Children's emotional manifestation scale: development and testing. *Journal of Clinical Nursing* 2003, 14: 223–9.

Ho Han J, Hwa Park S, Sam Lee B, Un Choi S. Erect penile size of Korean men. *Venereology* 1999, 12(14): 135–9.

Hosmer DW, Lemeshow S. *Applied Logistic Regression*. Chichester: John Wiley, 1989.

Hosmer DW, Lemeshow S (1999). *Applied Survival Analysis*. Chichester: John Wiley & Sons., Ltd.

Hundley V, Milne J, Leighton-Beck L, Graham W, Fitzmaurice A. Raising research awareness among midwives and nurses: does it work? *Journal of Advanced Nursing* 2000, 31: 78–88.

Jernström H, Olsson H. Breast size in relation to endogenous hormone levels, body constitution, and oral contraceptive use in healthy nulligravid women aged 19–25 years. *American Journal of Epidemiology* 1997, 45: 571–80.

Judge K, Benzeval M. Health inequalities: new concerns about the children of single mothers. *BMJ* 1993, 306: 677–80.

Kong S. Day treatment programme for patients with eating disorders: randomized controlled trial. *Journal of Advanced Nursing* 2005, 51(1): 5–14.

Kremer C, Duffy S, Moroney M. Patient satisfaction with outpatient hysteroscopy versus day case hysteroscopy: randomised controlled trial. *BMJ* 2000, 320: 279 82.

Kroman N, Jensen M-B, Wohlfahrt J, Mouridsen HT, Andersen PK, Melbye M. Factors influencing the effect of age on prognosis in breast cancer: population based study. *BMJ* 2000, 320: 474–9.

Kwakkel G, Wagenaar RC, Twisk JWR, Lankhorst GJ, Koetsier JC. Intensity of leg and arm training after primary middle-cerebral-artery stroke: a randomised trial. *Lancet* 1999, 354: 191–6.

Lacy AM, Garcia-Valdecasas JC, Delgado S, Castells A, Taura P, Pique JM, Visa J. Laparoscopy-assisted colectomy versus open colectomy for treatment of non-metastastic colon cancer: a randomised trial. *Lancet* 2002, 359: 2224–9.

Ledergerber B, Egger M, Opravil M, *et al.* Clinical progression and virological failure on highly active antiretroviral therapy in HIV-1 patients: a prospective cohort study. *Lancet* 1999, 353: 863–8.

Levene S. More injuries from 'bouncy castles'. *BMJ* 1992, 304: 1311–12.

Lien J, Chan V. Risk factors influencing survival in acute renal failure treated by hemodialysis. *Archives of Internal Medicine* 1985, 45: 2067–9.

Lin L-C, Wang TG, Chen MY, Wu SC, Portwood MJ. Depressive symptoms in long-term care residents in Taiwan. *Journal of Advanced Nursing* 2005, 51: 30–7.

Lindelow M, Hardy R, Rodgers B. Development of a scale to measure symptoms of anxiety and depression in the general UK population: the psychiatric symptom frequency scale. *Journal of Epidemiology and Community Health* 1997, 51: 549–57.

Little P. GP documentation of obesity: what does it achieve? *British Journal of General Practice* 1998, 48: 890–4.

Little P, Williamson I, Warner G, Gould C, Gantley M, Kinmonth AL. Open randomised trial of prescribing strategies in managing sore throat. *BMJ* 1997, 314: 722–7.

Long EM, Martin HL, Kriess JK, Rainwater SMJ, Lavreys L, Jackson DJ, Rakwar J, Mandaliya K, Overbaugh J. Gender differences in HIV-1 diversity at time of infection. *Nature Medicine* 2000, 6: 71–5.

Macarthur A, Macarthur C, Weeks S. Epidural anaesthesia and low back pain after delivery: a prospective cohort study. *BMJ* 1995, 311: 1336–9.

Mansi JL, Gogas H, Bliss JM, Gazet JC, Berger U, Coombes RC. Outcome of primary-breast-cancer patients with micrometastases: a long-term follow-up study. *Lancet* 1999, 354: 197–202.

Marshall M, Lockwood A, Gath D. Social services case-management for long-term mental disorders: a randomised controlled trial. *Lancet* 1995, 345: 409–12.

McKee M, Hunter D. Mortality league tables: do they inform or mislead? *Quality in Health Care* 1995, 4: 5–12.

McKeown-Eyssen GE, Sokoloff ER, Jazmaji V, Marshall LM, Baines CJ. Reproducibility of the University of Toronto self-administered questionnaire used to assess environmental sensitivity. *American Journal of Epidemiology* 2000, 151: 1216–22.

Merit-HF Study Group. Effect of metoprolol CR/XL in chronic heart failure: Metoprolol CR/XL Randomised Intervention Trial in Congestive Heart Failure (MERIT-HF). *Lancet* 1999, 353: 2001–7.

Michelson D, Stratakis C, Hill L, Reynolds J, Galliven E, Chrousos G, Gold P. Bone mineral density in women with depression. *NEJM* 1996, 1176–80.

Miles K, Penny N, Power R, Mercy D. Comparing doctor- and nurse-led care in sexual health clinics: patient satisfaction questionnaire. *Journal of Advanced Nursing* 2002, 42: 64–72.

Moore RA, Tramèr MR, Carroll D, Wiffen PJ, McQuay HJ. Quantitative systematic review of topically applied non-steroidal anti-inflammatory drugs, *BMJ* 1998, 316: 333–8.

Morris CR, Kato GJ, Poljakovic M, Wang X, Blackwelder WC, Sachdev V, Hazen SL, Vichinsky EP, Morris SM, Gladwin MT. Dysregulated arginine metabolism, hemolysis-associated pulmonary hypertension, and mortality in sickle cell disease. *Journal of the American Medical Association* 2005, 294: 81–90.

Möttönen T, Hannonen P, Leirisalo-Repo M, *et al.* Comparison of combination therapy with single-drug therapy in early rheumatoid arthritis: a randomised trial. *Lancet* 1999, 353: 1568–73.

Murray E, Jolly B, Modell M. Can students learn clinical methods in general practice? A randomised crossover trial based on objective structured clinical examinations. *BMJ* 1997, 315: 920–3.

Naumburg E, Bellocco R, Cnattingius S, Hall P, Ekbom A. Prenatal ultrasound examinations and risk of childhood leukaemia: case-control study. *BMJ* 2000, 320: 282–3.

Nead KG, Halterman JS, Kaczorowski JM, Auinger P, Weitzman M. Overweight children and adolescents: a risk group for iron deficiency. *Pediatrics* 2004, 114: 104–8.

Nikolajsen L, Ilkjaer S, Christensen JH, Krøner K, Jensen TS. Randomised trial of epidural bupivacaine and morphine in prevention of stump and phantom pain in lower-limb amputation. *Lancet* 1998, 350: 1353–7.

Oliver D, Britton M, Seed P, Martin FC, Hopper AH. Development and evaluation of evidence based risk assessment tool (STRATIFY) to predict which elderly inpatients will fall: case–control and cohort studies. *BMJ* 1997, 315: 1049–53.

Olson J, Shu XO, Ross JA, Pendergrass T, Robison LL. Medical record validation of maternally reported birth characteristics and pregnancy-related events: a report from the Children's Cancer Group. *American Journal of Epidemiology* 1997, 145(1): 58–67.

Peabody JW, Gertler PJ. Are clinical criteria just proxies for socioeconomic status? A study of low birth weight in Jamaica. *Journal of Epidemiology and Community Health* 1997, 51: 90–5.

Phipatanakul W, Celedon JC, Raby BA, Litonjua AA, Milton DK, Sredl D, Weiss ST, Gold DR. Endotoxin exposure and eczema in the first year of life. *Pediatrics* 2004, 114: 13–18.

Pinnock H, Bawden R, Proctor S, Wolfe S, Scullion J, Price D, Sheikh A. Accessibility, acceptability, and effectiveness in primary care of routine telephone review of asthma: pragmatic, randomised controlled trial. *BMJ* 2003, 326: 477–9.

Pisacane A, Sansone R, Impagliazzo N, *et al.* Iron deficiency anaemia and febrile convulsions: case–control study in children under 2 years. *BMJ* 1996, 313: 343.

Platt S, Tannahill A, Watson J, Fraser E, Effectiveness of antismoking telephone helpline: follow up survey. *BMJ* 1997, 314: 1371–5.

Pollack IF, Finkelstein SD, Woods J, Burnham J, Holmes EJ, Hamilton RL, Yates AJ, Boyett JM, Finlay JL, Sposto R. Expression of p53 and prognosis in children with malignant gliomas. *New England Journal of Medicine* 2002, 346: 420–7.

Poulter NR, Chang CL, MacGregor AJ, Snieder H, Spector TD. Association between birth weight and adult blood pressure in twins: historical cohort study. *BMJ* 1999, 319: 1330–3.

Premawardhena AP, de Silva CE, Fonseka MMD, Gunatilake SB, de Silva HJ. Low dose subcutaneous adrenaline to prevent acute adverse reactions to antivenom serum in people bitten by snakes: randomised, placebo controlled trial. *BMJ* 1999, 318: 1041–3.

Reidy A, Minassian DC, Vafidis G, *et al.* Prevalence of serious eye disease and visual impairment in a north London population: population based, cross sectional study. *BMJ* 1998, 316: 1643–6.

Rodgers M, Miller JE. Adequacy of hormone replacement therapy for osteoporosis prevention assessed by serum oestradiol measurement, and the degree of association with menopausal symptoms. *British Journal of General Practice* 1997, 47: 161–6.

Rogers SL, Farlow MR, Doody RS, Mohs R, Friedhoff LT, for the Donepezil Study Group. A 24-week, double-blind, placebo-controlled trial of donepezil in patients with Alzheimer's disease. *Neurology* 1998, 50: 136–45.

Salmon G, James A, Smith DM. Bullying in schools: self reported anxiety, depression, and self esteem in secondary school children. *BMJ* 1998, 317: 924–5.

Singer G, Freedman LS. Injuries sustained on 'bouncy castles'. *BMJ* 1992, 304: 912.

Singh A, Crockard HA. Quantitative assessment of cervical spondylotic myelopathy by a simple walking test. *Lancet* 1999, 354: 370–3.

Smith D, Pearce L, Pringle M, Caplan R. Adults with a history of child sexual abuse: evaluation of a pilot therapy service. *BMJ* 1995, 310: 1175–8.

Søyseth V, Kongerud J, Haarr D, Strand O, Bolle R, Boe J. Relation of exposure to airway irritants in infancy to prevalence of bronchial hyper-responsiveness in schoolchildren. *Lancet* 1995, 345: 217–20.

Streiner DL, Norman GR (1995). *Health Measurement Scales: A Practical Guide to their Development and Use*, Oxford: Oxford University Press.

Tang JL, Armitage JM, Lancaster T, Silagy CA, Fowler GH, Neil HAW. Systematic review of dietary intervention trials to lower blood total cholesterol in free-living subjects. *BMJ* 1998, 316: 1213–9.

Taylor DW, Barnett HJM, Haynes RB, *et al.* Low-dose and high-dose acetylsalicylic acid for patients undergoing carotid endarterectomy: a randomised controlled trial. *Lancet* 1999, 353: 2179–84.

Tebartz van Elst L, Woermann FG, Lemieux L, Thompson PJ, Trimble MR. Affective aggression in patients with temporal lobe epilepsy: a quantitative MRI study of the amygdala. *Brain* 2000, 123: 234–43.

Thompson C, Kinmonth AL, Stevens L, Peveler RC, Stevens A, Ostler KJ, Pickering RM, Baker NG, Henson A, Preece J, Cooper D, Campbell MJ. Effects of a clinical-practice guideline and practice-based education on detection and outcome of depression in primary care: Hampshire Depression Project randomised controlled trial. *Lancet* 2000, 355: 185–9.

Topol EJ, Ferguson JJ, Weisman HF, Tcheng JE, Ellis SG, Kleiman NS, Ivanhoe RJ, Wang AL, Miller DP, Anderson KM, Califs RM for the EPIC Investigator Group Long-term protection from myocardial ischaemic events in a randomized trial of brief integrin β_3 blockade with percutaneous coronary intervention. *JAMA* 1997, 278: 479–84.

Turnbull D, Holmes A, Shields N, Cheyne H, Twaddle S, Gilmour WH, McGinley M, Reid M, Johnstone I, Geer I, McIlwaine G, Lunan CB. Randomised, controlled trial of efficacy of midwife-managed care. *Lancet* 1996, 348: 213–18.

Unwin C, Blatchley N, Coker W, Fery S, Hotopf M, Hull L, Ismail K, Palmer I, David A, Wessley S. Health of UK servicemen who served in the Persian Gulf War. *Lancet* 1999, 353: 169–78.

Van Steirteghem AC, Zweig MH, Robertson EA, Bernard RM, Putzeys GA, Bieva CJ. Comparison of the effectiveness of four clinical chemical assays in classifying patients with chest pain. *Clinical Chemistry* 1982, 28: 1319–24.

Wald NJ, Law MR, Morris JK, Bagnall AM. *Helicobacter pylori* infection and mortality from ischaemic heart disease: negative result from a large, prospective study. *BMJ* 1997, 315: 1199–201.

Index

Understanding Clinical Papers Second Edition   David Bowers, Allan House, David Owens
© 2006 John Wiley & Sons, Ltd